FEED ZONE
TABLE

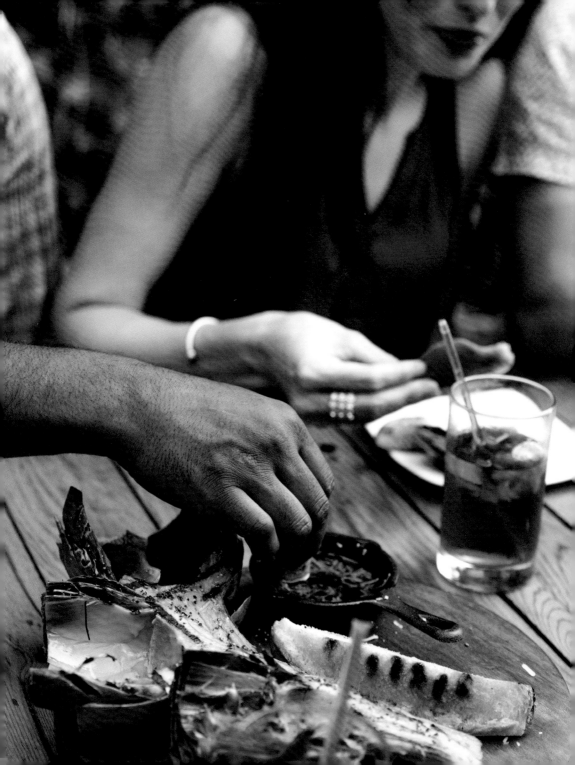

FEED ZONE
TABLE

FAMILY-STYLE MEALS
TO NOURISH LIFE AND SPORT

BIJU THOMAS & ALLEN LIM

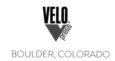

BOULDER, COLORADO

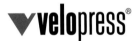

3002 Sterling Circle, Suite 100
Boulder, Colorado 80301-2338 USA
(303) 440-0601 ★ Fax (303) 444-6788
velopress@competitorgroup.com

Distributed in the United States and Canada
by Ingram Publisher Services

A Cataloging-in-Publication record for this book is available
from the Library of Congress.
ISBN 978-1-937715-40-3

For information on purchasing VeloPress books,
please call (800) 811-4210 ext. 2138 or visit www.velopress.com.

16 17 18 / 10 9 8 7 6 5 4 3 2 1

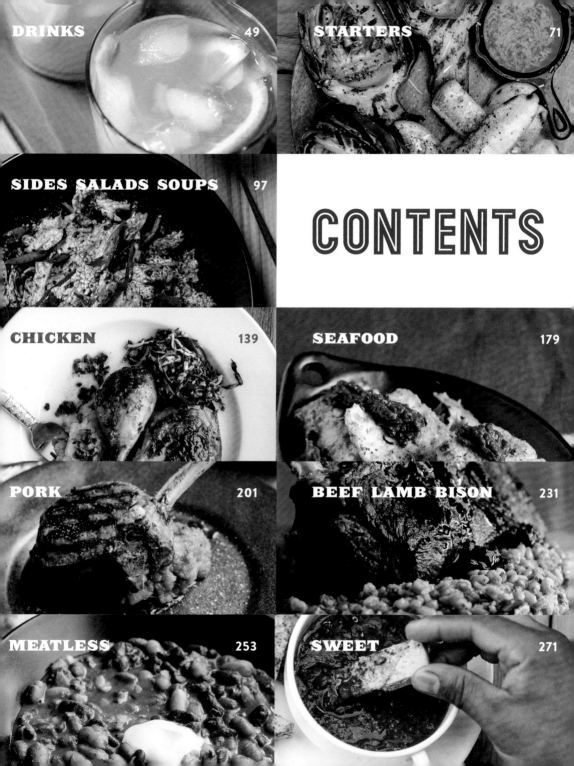

CONTENTS

DRINKS 49

STARTERS 71

SIDES SALADS SOUPS 97

CHICKEN 139

SEAFOOD 179

PORK 201

BEEF LAMB BISON 231

MEATLESS 253

SWEET 271

Foreword   **xi**
Preface   **xv**

Introduction   Where to Sit **1** · Social Fuel **3** · Five-Ring Fever **5** ·
                    Copernican Shift **8** · Eating Together **11** · Head Count **13** ·
                    Diet-Health Paradox **17** · Loneliness **21** · "We" Versus "I" **28**
                    · Cultural Dilemma **30** · Nutritional Pragmatism **35** ·
                    The Last Word **40**

Recipes   Eat & Cook **43**

DRINKS   Lemon Hibiscus Iced Tea with Honey   **52**
                    Mumbai Spiced Chai   **55**
                    Spiced Apple Cider   **56**
                    Salty Cucumber Lime Soda   **59**
                    Watermelon Soda with Fresh Mint   **60**
                    Vietnamese-Style Coffee   **62**
                    Sparkling Ginger Soda   **64**
                    Swiss Mountain Herb Tea   **66**
                    Homemade Hot Chocolate   **69**

STARTERS   Grilled Bread & Artichokes with Dipping Oil   **73**
                    Guacamole with Beans   **77**
                    Italian Rice Balls with Red Pepper Oil & Lemon Pesto **78**
                    White Anchovy Toast   **83**
                    Toasted Chickpeas with Ghost Pepper Salt   **84**
                    Tuna Mushroom Salad with Lemon Tarragon Dressing **87**
                    Bitter Chard on Grilled Bread   **88**
                    Classic Hummus   **91**

SIDES   Chilled Black Bean Yogurt Soup   **102**
SALADS   Turkey Meatball & Tomato Soup   **105**
SOUPS   Torn Bread & Radicchio Salad   **106**
                    Chile & Lime–Spiced Bay Scallops   **108**
                    Olive Oil–Poached Tomato Soup with Walnuts   **110**
                    Fresh Grapefruit & Avocado Salad   **113**

Coconut Rice Porridge with Adacherri		**115**
Broccoli Soup with Smoked Trout & Chives		**117**
Spicy Red Beans & Rice		**118**
Sweet Potato–Stuffed Wonton Soup		**121**
Grilled Romaine with Pancetta, Hard-Boiled Eggs & Dijon Dressing		**123**
Kimchee Spiced Salad		**127**
Citrus Salad with Yuzu Dressing & Wonton Crisps		**128**
Warm German Potato Salad		**131**
Pan-Roasted Chickpeas & Summer Vegetables		**132**
Pasta with Maple Carrots & Leeks		**135**
Cauliflower & Corn Chowder with Red Pepper Oil		**137**
CHICKEN	Rustic Lemon Chicken	**140**
	Masala Chicken Wrap with Cabbage Slaw	**143**
	Kalamata Chicken with New Potatoes	**144**
	Chopped Chicken Salad with Pickled Onions & Radishes	**147**
	Baked Chicken Parmesan with Bright & Chunky Marinara	**149**
	Split Chicken with Lemon Garlic Sauce & Roasted Vegetables	**154**
	Chicken Pad Thai	**156**
	Sautéed Tortellini & Sausage with Collard Greens	**158**
	Grilled Chicken with Homemade Barbecue Sauce	**160**
	Chicken & Almond Dumplings	**165**
	Chicken Madras & Yogurt Sauce with Harissa	**166**
	Red Chicken with Baked Biriyani	**170**
SEAFOOD	Baked Jambalaya	**180**
	Catfish Piccata	**183**
	Grilled Salmon Steak Sandwiches	**184**
	Miso & Maple–Marinated Cod with Sweet Pea Risotto	**186**
	Baked Salmon in Pastry	**191**
	Lobster Mac 'n' Cheese with Fresh Tomatillo Sauce	**193**
	Pepper-Crusted Cod with Sambal	**196**
	Ginger Barbecue Salmon	**198**

PORK

Sausage, Potato & Kale Soup	203
Grilled Pork Chops with Kabocha Squash Mash	204
Blackened Pork Loin & Pickled Onions with Baked Apples	208
Stewed Black-Eyed Peas with Salt Pork	213
Santa Fe Mac 'n' Cheese	215
Roast Pork Loin with Peach Glaze & White Beans	216
Country-Style Hoisin Ribs	219
Allen's Ramen	221

BEEF LAMB BISON

Flank Steak with Torn Heirloom Tomatoes	233
Beef & Beet Meatloaf	235
Irish Lamb Stew with Guinness & Soda Bread	237
Mac 'n' Cheese Bolognese	241
Bison Stew with Barley & Belgian Beer	243
Grilled T-Bones with Blue Cheese Dressing & Radicchio Slaw	245
Lamb Chops with Cherry Jam, Farro & Fennel Slaw	248

MEATLESS

Chilled Soba with Spicy Red Beans & Poached Eggs	254
Baked Ziti with Toasted Chickpeas & Squash	257
Mixed Bean Curry	259
Falafel with Chunky Cucumber Yogurt Sauce	262
Sweet Potato, Pecan & Mushroom "Meatloaf"	265
Eggplant & Onion Fried Wild Rice	266
Homemade Egg Pasta with Fresh-Chopped Sauce	269

SWEET

Banana Mousse Dessert	272
PB&J Cookies	275
Cashew Honey Brittle	277
Baked Granola Crisp	278
Almond Cornbread with Grilled Stone Fruit	281
Dark Chocolate Bark with Spiced Pumpkin Seeds	282
Baklava	285
Cinnamon Shortbread Cookies with Fresh Jam	287

Oils & Dressings

Balsamic Dipping Oil **73** · Red Pepper Oil **78** · Lemon Tarragon Dressing **87** · Dijon Dressing **123** · Red Pepper Sesame Oil Dressing **127** · Yuzu Dressing **128** · Mustard Yogurt Dressing **184** · Blue Cheese Dressing **245**

Sauces & Spices

Lemon Pesto **80** · Ghost Pepper Salt Mix **84** · Adacherri **115** · Bright & Chunky Marinara **149** · Lemon Garlic Sauce **154** · Homemade Barbecue Sauce **163** · Yogurt Sauce **166** · Harissa **168** · Roasted Tomato Yogurt Sauce **172** · Roux **180** · Fresh Tomatillo Sauce **195** · Sambal **196** · Ginger Barbecue Sauce **198** · Basic Grilling Salt **206** · Vindaloo Spice Mix **209** · Fresh Jalapeño Hot Sauce **215** · Hoisin Sauce **219** · Cherry Jam **248** · Chunky Cucumber Yogurt Sauce **262** · Fresh-Chopped Sauce **269**

Nutrition Facts   293
Notes   299
Index   306
Acknowledgments   314
About the Authors   316
Credits   318

FOREWORD

In another life, I raced bikes for a living. As with any professional sport, many people go to great lengths to make the dream a reality. They push in all their chips for that jackpot. For me, becoming a pro cyclist was more of a happy accident. I was a distance runner and an All-American in the indoor mile, and a three-time All-American in the 3000-meter steeplechase during college. I was injured near the end of my career, and with my enthusiasm match spent, I became a garbage man. And I rode my bike . . . a lot. I joined a local Colorado team, did a few big races, and even won a big one down in New Mexico. I realized that I had a chance to do something special in cycling. Because I didn't have anything to lose and it sounded fun, when I got the call from a pro cycling team, I took that chance. I signed for Garmin-Slipstream in 2007 and hopped on a plane to Europe.

I showed up at my first training camp and looked around at my new teammates. We all shared simple goal—to ride our bikes faster, especially when it counts—in a race. For the team or any one individual to succeed, we all needed to ride hard and race harder.

Even though our team dinners were a place where most riders gathered to eat and unwind from a hard day of training or racing, for me they led to a dysfunctional relationship with food. I couldn't stop comparing what was on my plate to what my teammates were eating. I figured they had more experience with racing and fueling, so I should probably eat like they did. Humans are social creatures who like to be accepted by their tribe, and this can lead to a real conundrum for someone who is trying to prove himself on a world stage.

Being a pro comes with benefits, the kind we all talk about, but the sheer force of that drive to be faster can be isolating. Most of the time it's just you and that guy next to you, riding in the gutter, teeth clenched, dirty, hurting, tired, scared, and hungry. Even though I was surrounded by a bunch of guys with the same goals as me, I was really eating alone at our team meals. The questions weighed heavily

When I eat a meal with people I love, the experience meets a deep-seated need that goes well beyond my body's need for carbohydrates, protein, and fat.

on my mind. It really didn't matter how healthy the food was that I chose to eat, it wasn't doing much for me, or my performance. Over time I came to the realization that those questions about fueling were influencing my training decisions negatively, and I eventually lost my place on the team.

While my pro cycling career was short-lived, I did make a few solid impressions. I made my debut as a pro at the 2007 Tour of California and finished second to Levi Leipheimer in the first stage, much to everyone's shock. I also won a stage at the Tour of Utah in 2008. Most of the time, I rode in support of our team leaders, controlling the pace at the front of the pack so a teammate could ride for the win. That first big day in 2007 defined my career—I was the inexperienced guy with a big engine. Ultimately, I lacked confidence in my abilities as an athlete and in my preparation.

While I was racing on the pro circuit, I did learn a lot about food and my relation-ship with it. Europeans love their food and the traditions that surround it. I grew to love my food too, but it took a while. When I retired from cycling, I started cooking for real. It was a task I took on somewhat begrudgingly, but I decided that if this was something that I had to do every day, I was going to do it right. Somewhere along the way I learned to love cooking. I began inviting friends over for dinner. I wasn't making anything fancy—I was just turning simple, fresh, familiar foods into a home-cooked meal. The warm conversation and laughter of my friends and family gathered in anticipation of a meal has given me one of the most satisfying feelings I know.

These days my family is my first priority. Both my wife and I work full time, and we have two young kids to raise. Most days I walk in the door after a day at the office and head straight into the kitchen to cook dinner. It gives me a great sense of purpose. I want my children to know the nourishing power of a home-cooked meal. When I eat a meal with people I love, the experience meets a deep-seated need that goes well beyond my body's need for carbohydrates, protein, and fat.

I work with Allen at Skratch Labs, and every Wednesday morning promptly at 8 a.m. we sit down to a home-cooked breakfast with our team. Whether we are commiserating or celebrating, those breakfasts go down as some of the best-tasting, most nourishing meals I have eaten.

It's ironic that today, as I attempt to balance family, work, and sport, my athletic performance is as good as it has ever been. All of the metrics, including my age, are less favorable than they were when I was racing in Europe. But one thing is clearly different—I sit down to home-cooked meals on a regular basis now. I cook for my family and my friends at every opportunity. Skratch Labs is even supporting me as I begin training in a more focused way for cyclocross and trail running. For me, the adventure is far from over. Perhaps it's only just begun.

Use the recipes in this book to test the impact of a home-cooked meal for yourself. Don't eat alone—include your friends and family in the experiment. Give it time, and I'm confident you will enjoy results, both at the table and in your sport.

JASON DONALD
Former pro cyclist & All-American runner
Director of Stoke, Skratch Labs
Father, husband, athlete

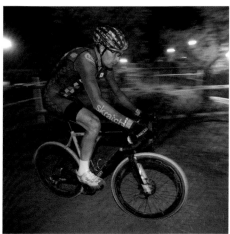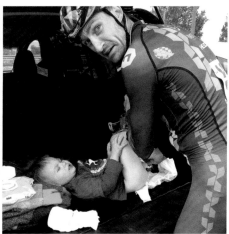

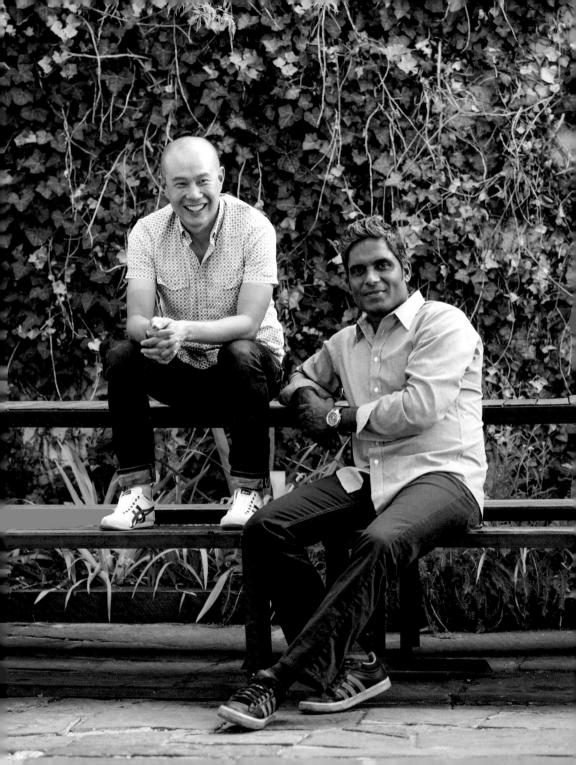

PREFACE

Chef Biju and I wrote *The Feed Zone Cookbook* and *Feed Zone Portables* for anyone interested in improving athletic performance. So when we heard that people who don't necessarily consider themselves athletes were using our cookbooks because they wanted simple, healthy recipes to share with their friends and family, we were pleasantly surprised . . . and inspired.

We've always believed that physical activity and sport are central to our individual and cultural health. More important, we know that proper nutrition is fundamental to supporting an athletic lifestyle. But for us, neither sport nor nutrition is solely about performance. The reality is that we value activity and food not just because we want to perform better but also because both have this amazing ability to bring people together, to give us pleasure, and to feed our souls. How we gather and share on a human level is at the very heart of what makes us happy and healthy. And if there's anything we've learned from sport and life, it's our happiness and health that drive performance and success, not our performance or success that make us happy or healthy.

We are not interested in perpetuating the idea that there has to be a certain way that athletes eat for performance that is somehow different from how nonathletes eat for health and well-being.

With that in mind, *Feed Zone Table* is our acknowledgment that we are our happiest and best when we find community with one another. This book is a thank-you to everyone who's ever told us that our cookbooks have brought their families closer together, as well as encouragement and applause for those who are willing to make the effort to get themselves, their friends, their kids, their parents, or their teammates into the kitchen to cook.

**For the athletes we know and love,
this book is a resource to help bolster the fragile line
separating athletic drive from isolation.**

While we all intuitively know that recipes made from scratch that use fresh, whole foods are the best for our health and performance, it's equally important to recognize that coming together with others for a meal often drives us to prepare healthier foods. In the same way that it's hard to talk about nutrition without talking about food, it's hard to talk about food without talking about people and their influence on how and what we eat. Like the magic stone that makes stone soup, the real secret is not a single ingredient but collaboration—setting aside our own self-interest, even for a moment, to care for and cook with others.

Obviously, there are differences between how an elite athlete might eat versus someone who is only moderately active or even sedentary. Portion size or the relative amount of macronutrients such as carbohydrate and fat, for example, will differ for different people. And certainly, *The Feed Zone Cookbook* and *Feed Zone Portables* take an athlete-centric approach to eating and cooking. But, as proud as we are of those cookbooks, we are not interested in perpetuating the idea that there has to be a certain way that athletes eat for performance that is somehow different from how nonathletes eat for health and well-being. Even if individuals choose to build their plates differently, we know from experience that athletes and nonathletes can eat from the same table. The problem is, we see more and more people so caught up in the pursuit of performance that they end up eating alone, in part because they define their nutritional needs as distinct from others, including their very close friends, family, and teammates. What we want is for people to share—to be inclusive rather than exclusive.

It's taken a lot of time to develop this perspective. When I first left the rigors of academia to practice the craft of sport science, I had this romantic vision that I was going to be working to uncover marginal gains—the tiny details and innovation that would keep athletes on the winning side of the exceptionally small margin between success and failure.

Unfortunately, I entered into a dysfunctional culture so focused on the science of performance that fundamentals were being ignored and becoming bottlenecks. Coursing through the world of elite cycling, the sport I chose as my professional focus, was a gold vein of potential fueled by young athletes who lacked the basic life skills they needed to take care of themselves and each other. They were adult children. Instead of legends and giants, I found people disconnected from their homes, families, and friends, trying to perform their best under an enormous amount of pressure. Despite being part of a team, these remarkably talented athletes in the prime of their lives spent a significant amount of their time alone and lonely. Athletes will gladly go to extremes with their training and diet, all in the name of performance. The sad reality, however, is that too often the goal of performance pushes athletes into a withdrawn lifestyle that is innately selfish and isolating. Trying to manage a sport-specific diet can add to that isolation.

For the athletes we know and love, this book is a resource to help bolster the fragile line separating athletic drive from isolation. While it's often the case that we use our pursuit of sport as an escape, real nourishment—the kind we get from sharing a meal with those we care for—may very well be the ingredient we need most as we push ourselves to be and perform better. This book is a reminder that we don't have to hide behind our ambition or sport—that we can actually accomplish more if we view our nutrition as nourishment shared in the company of others. This isn't just touchy-feely sentiment. There is strong scientific evidence demonstrating that the context of a meal can both shape the meal itself as well as our psychological and physiological response to it. Simply put, regardless of the meal, we do better when we consistently eat with others, and we do worse when we mostly eat alone.

It's with all of this in mind that we return to the kitchen for what we consider the most social meal of the day—dinner. No matter how you define family, we sincerely hope that the ideas and recipes in this cookbook create a deeper foundation for family-style meals as a basic life skill and habit. Like all of our cookbooks, this isn't about following every instruction to the letter, counting grams, or solving the world's problems. It's about using fresh, whole ingredients, tasting, modifying, and having fun. Cooking is rarely a perfect process. But it is a process—one that does not have to be a solitary chore, one that continuously evolves as we learn, and one that has its own reward and joy. Ultimately, *Feed Zone Table* is our way of sharing and inspiring simple, healthy, and performance-driven dinners that bring great food and people to the table. Because no matter what our size, speed, goal, or disposition, we all thrive when we play, cook, and eat together.

INTRODUCTION

There is strong scientific evidence demonstrating that the context of a meal can both shape the meal itself as well as our psychological and physiological response to it.

WHERE TO SIT

The very first professional bicycle race I worked at in Europe was the Volta a Catalunya in northern Spain in 2005. That race was an uncomfortable lesson in the intricacies of etiquette and tradition in European cycling, and as an outsider I didn't fare too well.

What I didn't know then was that at dinner-time during a stage race, the tradition is that the riders all sit at one table while the staff sit at another. Although it is, in my opinion, an outdated version of the kids' versus adults' table, it was nonetheless the norm.

So at my first "professional" dinner, with a full plate of food gathered from the hotel buffet, I found myself *not knowing where to sit*. It was absolutely clear I wasn't a rider, but I was far from being accepted as staff. Not knowing where to go, I regressed into my clumsy 12-year-old self on the first day of middle school as I looked for somewhere to put myself in this foreign cafeteria, which could have doubled for a very bad version of a Disney cruise ship. Realizing that the staff was not welcoming me, Floyd Landis abruptly pulled up an extra chair at the riders' table and told me to sit, if only to calm the intense awkwardness of the situation as I stood there like a deer in headlights. I didn't belong. This wasn't my tribe, and I had a lot to prove.

Later that year, I began to find my stride, but not with the Europeans. Instead, it was with a group of juniors and under-23 cyclists on the TIAA-CREF development team. Unlike the Pro Tour teams, at races there was little separation between athletes and staff in our motley crew of mostly young Americans. Although there was a designated athletes' table and staff table, the lines weren't closely followed. We were very much a big family. Less time was spent eating than joking, laughing, and sharing stories of the day. Race meals were like summer camp. But teaching a group of very young, talented athletes how to take care of themselves when they were on their own was a different story—a story that formed the basic motivation for the cooking experiments and recipes shared in *The Feed Zone Cookbook*.

As that young TIAA-CREF development squad slowly matured and developed into the Garmin Professional Cycling Team, our team dinners evolved too. At our very first Tour de France, in 2008, Christian Vande Velde, the team captain, was adamant that all of the riders be present at the dinner table before anyone started eating. As a kid there were few things that got Christian in as much trouble as missing a family dinner. And at the Tour, the team was our family and he was our leader, so his sense of family tradition reigned. While we still joked, told stories, and laughed, Christian's "rule" ensured that people were on time and created an atmosphere of mutual respect, elevating the importance of what our team dinners represented. Dinner was a time to commune, to take comfort by reflecting on the day with people who understood the madness of our situation, and a way to regain both the mental and physical strength to do it all again. It was the only calm we had each day—a sanctuary where nobody was ever worried about where to sit.

What these team dinners reinforced is that food isn't just a source of fuel, as it often seems to be during training and

HUMAN PERFORMANCE

competition. It's also a source of belonging. Food is part of what Abraham Maslow described as a "hierarchy of needs."[1] At the bottom of that hierarchy are our basic physiological needs, which include our primal urge to satiate hunger and thirst. Those physiological requirements are followed by our need for safety and

Food isn't just a source of fuel, as it often seems to be during training and competition. It's also a source of belonging.

security. Third on the hierarchy is our need to belong—a need that falls even before our need for self-esteem and self-actualization. We often associate success in sport, work, and life with the top of Maslow's hierarchy—the esteem and self-actualization that come from being our very best. But without a foundation of food, shelter, and belonging, it's difficult to realize any of those higher personal goals. Thus, it is as important to mind what we eat as it is to eat in a way that fosters intimacy and connection with one another. Making the effort to do so may not always be convenient, easy, or even comfortable, but that doesn't change the fact that it is a critical and essential part of being human. If there's anything I learned during my work on the Pro Cycling Tour, it's that when all is said and done, it's the *human* part of the human performance equation that really matters.

SOCIAL FUEL

As infants and children we rely entirely on others for food, shelter, and, most important, love. Not only are we given a life through this care, but we inherit—if we choose to accept it—a culture. We gain a social structure that can be as cultivated or as arbitrary as the food we eat.

It goes without saying that without adequate nutrition, people, especially young children, can become sick and even die, but many contend that inadequate love or attention can have even grimmer consequences. Mutually beneficial care and nurturing is what psychologist Monte Atkinson refers to as "social fuel." Although our need for food is a given, social fuel may very well be as important as chemical fuel.

In Maslow's hierarchy of needs, belonging is described as essential but less important than our need for food, water, and security. As logical as this may sound, a series of infamous experiments by Harry Harlow brought into question the idea of a rigid linear hierarchy, demonstrating the fluidity and importance of all human needs.

In his research, Harlow conducted horrific isolation and maternal separation experiments on rhesus monkeys. He devised abusive strategies to disrupt the social structure innate to their rearing behavior, in some cases isolating infant monkeys for up to two years at a time. In all of these abnormal scenarios, the monkeys became severely disturbed, suffering in ways that many animal rights activists considered worse than death. In one particular set of studies, Harlow sought to understand the relationship between food and nurturing by creating two inanimate surrogate mothers—one covered in wire and one covered in cloth. When a bottle of food was placed with the wire surrogate, the monkeys would only engage with the wire surrogate to feed, but spent the rest of their time with the cloth-covered mother. And when some monkeys were provided with only a wire surrogate and not a cloth surrogate, those monkeys became sick, suffering from severe gastrointestinal distress despite gaining weight similar to the monkeys fed by the cloth surrogates. Though probably not intended as a cynical title, this work on the effects of cruelty and isolation was first published in a journal article called "The Nature of Love."[2] Still, Harlow's work demonstrated that while mere survival may have a hierarchal basis dependent first and foremost on food and water, the factors determining health and well-being are not so simple. Taken as a whole, the suffering and illness experienced by these animals demonstrated that food and water are not enough. Emotional needs cannot be neglected.

Sadly, it's unlikely that human infants would have survived the same treatment as Harlow's monkeys—a fact that was established well before either Harry Harlow or Abraham Maslow began thinking about human need.

Although our need for food is a given, social fuel may very well be as important as chemical fuel.

Just over a hundred years ago, a pediatrician named Dr. Henry Dwight Chapin began studying orphaned and destitute infants, reporting an unimaginable 100 percent death rate in babies under the age of two when they were placed in institutions in several major U.S. cities.[3] Chapin described isolated babies in orphanages with an untreatable marasmus—whole-body wasting, typically due to severe malnutrition. In these cases no amount of food reversed the marasmus, and eventually most of the infants died of other complications, such as pneumonia. Chapin believed that the isolation resulting from institutionalizing the babies killed them. He observed that when babies received human nurturing and touch,

especially while feeding, they survived and thrived, so he pioneered a "boarding-out," or foster care program, in which orphaned babies were placed in private homes so they could be cared for within a family unit.[4] This was the forebear of modern-day foster care in the United States, and by the end of World War II the orphanage as an institution in the United States was almost completely abolished, as was the marasmus that accompanied it.[5]

However, even when children do survive institutionalized care in other countries, they don't tend to do well as adults. For example, in Russia, where orphanages remain, 33 percent of adults raised in these institutions find themselves homeless, 20 percent are convicted of a crime, and 10 percent commit suicide—figures that are far above the norm.[6] Negative outcomes, however, are not limited to individual countries. In an analysis of data from 75 different studies examining more than 3,800 children living in 19 different countries, children raised in orphanages had an IQ that was 20 points lower on average compared to those in foster care.[7] This broad array of social and psychological problems stemming from severe deficits in early parental care is often labeled as "attachment disorder." The difficult lesson here is that we are fragile creatures and the love and care we receive very early in life influences our lifelong physical and mental health.

FIVE-RING FEVER

Even at the highest level of sport, familial care and support is critical to success. Although teams can act as strong and powerful surrogate families, the sentimental saying "There's no place like home" is a critical pillar of athletic performance.

It was one of the first big lessons I learned as a coach—a piece of humble pie that left me with a few scars and a more humanistic perspective on athletics.

I missed the graduation ceremony for my master's degree because I was at a job interview with Roy Knickman, a legendary cyclist and one of my childhood heroes, who was heading up a brand-new resident training program for a group of 16- to 19-year-old cyclists at the U.S. Olympic Training Center in Colorado Springs. At the time, the training methodology and ideology at USA Cycling were still influenced by the remnants of the Cold War rivalry between the Soviet Union and the United States. State-of-the-art training was based on Eastern European periodization programs that employed very specific blocks of training. Each block progressively worked a different physiological system over the course of a well-thought-out season until deep layers of adaptation brewed into perfectly timed peak performances.

Or at least that was the theory. As part of this theory, it was thought that this very regimented program needed to begin in earnest with children, at as early an age as possible. Although the U.S. Olympic Committee was far from allowing full-time training camps for young children, it was willing to relocate a group of talented teenagers so they could live and train at the Olympic Training Center while attending a local school. Because of this, a position had opened up for a resident coach who would live with and supervise these athletes on a daily basis. Fortunately, missing my graduation paid off and I was offered the position—my dream job—at the still-tender age of 24.

From a scientific perspective, I really believed the program had merit. I believed that the only way American cyclists were going to be competitive with the rest of the world was to start riders off with supervised, structured, and science-based training as early as possible. It would be a living and breathing model of perfect preparation. We were going to wake up each morning and piss excellence. My attitude was spartan.

The day the athletes arrived and began moving into the dorms, I beamed with pride and excitement as we began the first step toward officially chasing the Olympic dream. The athletes were equally excited. They were proud and motivated. Their energy was palpable. As I visited the athletes in their concrete dorm rooms, we talked as they unpacked and settled in. Like most kids their age, they hung posters and pictures of their friends and family

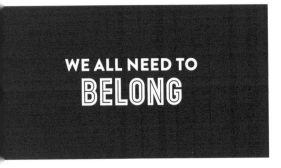

WE ALL NEED TO BELONG

on the wall. Unlike most teenagers, they also decorated their rooms with special mementos that reminded them of their extraordinary accomplishments and the spectacular opportunity ahead of them. Though they came from different parts of the country, at least a dozen athletes had been featured in local newspaper articles that celebrated their invitation to the Olympic Training Center. Those articles touted their talent and potential as future Olympians. A different article hung on each of the corkboards in almost every

dorm room. It was one of the first things to go up. With each athlete I met and each article I read, my excitement and pride grew exponentially.

A few weeks later, I began my daily routine of checking in with the athletes. As I walked from room to room, I noticed something was slightly different. At first, I wasn't quite sure what it was. But then it hit me. The newspaper articles were gone—and with them, the proof that each of these young athletes represented the very best from their local communities and the very best of what our country had to offer. Despite being some of the most talented athletes in the country, I think they began to feel that relative to everyone else they now lived and trained with, they weren't special anymore. Rather than focusing on the privilege and advantages associated with being national team athletes living and training at the epicenter of the U.S. Olympic Movement, they became focused on the competition, training load, and stress. Those local newspaper articles that started out as a source of pride and inspiration had become an embarrassment, and slowly they started coming down.

It was then that I realized the program wasn't going to work. We had inadvertently taken away from each of these athletes a key ingredient of their success to date. We had taken away their families and their friends. We took away the people who believed and cared for them the most:

When we tried to form a team, we instead fostered insecurity, because the basis of the group was the accomplishment of individual goals, not the betterment of a community. We put the need for personal success ahead of the need to belong.

their parents, siblings, teachers, childhood friends, and the community that gave its time, money, and love so they could reach their goals. Like Harlow's monkeys, forced to nurse from surrogate wire mothers, we had isolated these athletes. We put them in concrete rooms and fed them from a table made of five wire rings, hoping those wires—those Olympic rings—would be enough of a surrogate. The situation started making me feel sick. Instead of becoming stronger, most of the athletes became weaker. Similar to the children with unexplained marasmus whom Dr. Henry Chapin had observed during his visits to orphanages, these superhuman athletes were in essence becoming ill. So much so that we began calling the infectious disease the Olympic rings brought on "Five-Ring Fever." We wrongly assumed that America sends athletes to the Olympics, when in truth Americans do.

In my mind, those athletes are still some of the most gifted I have ever worked with. But slowly and surely the pressure, distance, and unfamiliar lifestyle we had imposed on them took its toll. Only one of those athletes would ever make it to the Olympic Games. In less than two years, the program was shelved, making room for older resident athletes, shorter-length training camps, and better-funded trips to Europe, where the experience of living and racing abroad could be practiced without permanently pulling kids away from their homes.

Although the resident training program was well intended, from the start we were going about it the wrong way. We put the need for personal success ahead of the need to belong. When we tried to form a team, we instead fostered insecurity, because the basis of the group was the accomplishment of individual goals, not the betterment of a community. These athletes weren't hunting for food to share with one another at the table, they were gunning for trophies to hang above their personal mantel. However, the real problem wasn't that personal happiness came before the team. It was that the goal of winning came before personal happiness. We fundamentally misjudged our orbit.

COPERNICAN SHIFT

When Nicolaus Copernicus proposed that the earth is actually in orbit around the sun instead of the sun orbiting around the earth, his "Copernican Shift" corrected a fundamental mistake about our place in the solar system and launched a scientific revolution. Dr. Shawn Achor, a psychologist who studies happiness, suggests that a similar paradigm shift is needed to improve our understanding of success and happiness.

Achor observes that most people wrongly believe success will bring them happiness. Unfortunately, accomplishing one goal only compels us to chase another, pushing happiness off indefinitely as we get caught in a never-ending pursuit. In contrast, when people find ways to be happy first, they become more creative, intelligent, energetic, and productive, which ultimately allows them to achieve more. The bottom line is that happiness does not revolve around success—success revolves around happiness.[8]

This simple idea applies to all facets of life, including sports, where we've been taught to fight, often against the tide, for what we feel or have been told we're entitled to. We think that hard work and sacrifice will drive achievement, so we embrace suffering as a badge of honor. Achievement alone, however, doesn't sustain the kind of long-term effort needed to be an athlete, or even to enjoy accomplishing a long-term goal.

In fact, postcompetition, a surprisingly large number of athletes become severely depressed after they cross the threshold of their pursuit.[9]

My observation has always been that athletes who have an unconditional and innate passion for their sport or activity are the most relentless and consistent. Not surprisingly, I also find that these athletes foster the unconditional support and care of others. These high achievers find much of their happiness outside of their ambition, in a close network of family and friends who they put, and who put them, ahead of their accomplishments. These athletes are secure in who they are, not just what they do. This sense of security and contentment fuels their performance. What happy and successful athletes teach us is that we are our best when we put people ahead of goals instead of goals ahead of people. We live in a culture personified by athletics, where we're taught to constantly push ourselves. The reality is that we just need to accept ourselves.

As someone who has built a career on giving people advice on how to push themselves harder, I regularly see this habit of putting success before happiness manifest as an obsession over what to eat. Even though I don't consider myself to

What happy and successful athletes teach us is that we are our best when we put people ahead of goals instead of goals ahead of people.

be a nutritionist, as a sport scientist the most common questions I am asked about performance revolve around food and the quest for the perfect diet.

Clearly, nutrition plays an undeniable role in athletic success and health. Unfortunately, when athletes ask me what to eat, rarely are they also considering who to eat with. They're worried about whether they are getting the perfect ratio of nutrients, not about taste, ingredients, or the positive social dynamics that manifest when sharing food. In fact, many athletes I know will gladly eat engineered prepackaged food by themselves if it means they can better meet whatever it is they believe to be their dietary goals. If one of the keys to real happiness is the unconditional bond we have with others,

then it's my belief that not being intentional about eating with others is the same as putting our notions of success ahead of our actual happiness or health.

It may be a stretch to say that who we eat with is more important than what we eat. But the more I think about what's backward about how we view nutrition, the more I believe that the act of sharing something as basic as our daily meals with others is the Copernican Shift we all need to recenter our approach to both sport and life. For as much time and energy as we put into perfecting our physical health or form, we put almost no time into our emotional or social health. After years of trying to help athletes be better, I've come to an extraordinarily simple epiphany that sharing a meal with others presents an invaluable opportunity to do both.

HAPPINESS vs. SUCCESS

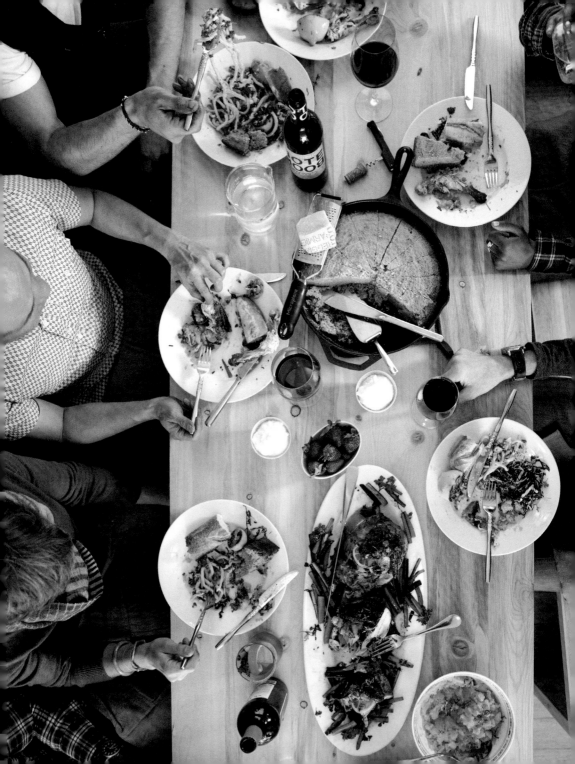

EATING TOGETHER

Given the integral link between our need for food and our need for others, it's hard to dispute the powerful psychological and physiological connection that comes from sitting down with one another for a meal.

While there may be a biological mechanism that explains the importance of eating with one another, the ritual of sharing a meal is as old as human history—an activity that has social and religious roots that predate our scientific understanding or interpretation.[10]

The act of eating and sharing food with one another is known as *commensality*, from the Latin *com* ("with") and *mensa* ("table"). More specifically, in Latin *mensa* is often used to describe a round table, connoting social equality.[11] The word *mensa* also has religious associations. In the Catholic faith, *mensa* is the stone slab that forms the top of the altar upon which the Holy Eucharist is performed, the ritual of transforming the symbolic body and blood of Jesus Christ into bread and wine to be shared during Communion.[12]

When humans first developed fire and began cooking and hunting with one another, we began sharing food together, which created a basic social order and structure through the allocation and distribution of essential resources. Many believe this is the very basis of economics,

religion, and modern-day government.[13] The sharing of food literally defines our participation in society. In fact, the word *participate* is originally derived from the Latin phrase *pars capere*, "share capture," which was used to describe people having their share of a sacrificial meal.[14]

From Roman banquets to Thanksgiving dinner, the ritual and tradition of coming together at a table to eat with one another touches almost every aspect of human civilization. Of note, commensality, like the complex societies we have built, is almost exclusively unique to humans. Outside of the act of nursing, no other animal has ever been observed actively sharing food with another except for the bonobo, which is our closest genetic relative.[15]

Today, the act of sharing food is one of the key social factors that we use to define friendship and intimacy. Eating together signals a positive and friendly social relationship, whereas feeding someone or being fed connotes a more familial or romantic relationship.[16] Intimacy and eating together are so tightly linked that for both men and women, learning that your romantic partner is eating with someone else sparks jealousy; however, hearing that your partner had a face-to-face interaction that doesn't involve eating doesn't elicit the same jealousy.[17]

If sport is nothing more than an artificial construct mimicking challenges of human survival from a distant past (like the hunting and gathering of food or protecting one another from wild animals or competing tribes), then pro cycling is the ultimate embodiment because it's the only sport in which teammates actively help shelter and feed one another. Within a frantic pack of cyclists racing down the road, there is a highly ordered system to accomplish the feeding process, which in turn dictates much of the activity in the peloton and the caravan of vehicles that follow behind it. Eating while racing a bike can be frenzied and brutish compared to sharing a meal at the dinner table, but for riders and staff, attending to those high-speed meals is one of the most important, laborious, and unifying aspects of the sport. Yet for all the energy and care spent feeding one another on the bike, I often hear complaints from these same athletes when off the bike between events about how difficult it is to either make time to eat with others or to find others to eat with.

This difficulty may be indicative of a greater social problem. As important as the sharing of food is to human nature, a moving peloton, and the very structure of our society, for the first time in human history there is concern that commensality is on a sharp decline. This showcases what some see as a growing tension between our individual versus collective nature, a conflict between our relatively recent sense of individual freedom and our age-old need to be part of a group.[18]

The very suggestion that commensality is on the decline threatens our ideation of the family meal. There's a sense that we are losing something that defines much of who we are, or at the very least who we think we are supposed to be.[19] Depending on the data set and the statistics, it's a concern that may be very well founded, with deeply negative social consequences. Or it may simply be another incarnation of moral panic—the feeling of fear, spreading like a contagion across a large group, that there is some apocalyptic threat to society.[20]

Whatever the cause and whatever the actual trend, one thing is clear—even within developed Western cultures where family structure and meals are thought to be most negatively affected, there is a high degree of variability when it comes to eating together. It's in this variability that we may be able to better understand whether eating together actually matters and whether we need to be worried if we find ourselves eating alone.

HEAD COUNT

One way to understand local and global cultural differences in commensality is to simply ask those who don't have much of a choice in the matter—our children.

When youths from different countries were asked how frequently most or all of those who lived in their household (i.e., family) sat down to eat together, the results varied greatly depending on factors such as region and income.

In the United States, some studies show that only 45–50 percent of youths report eating with their family or people they live with at what's considered to be a high frequency—five or more times per week.[21] That said, depending upon how the question is asked, there may be a great deal of variability. For example, in a group of 7,784 girls and 6,647 boys ages 9–14 who were surveyed across 50 states, 16 percent reported having family dinner "never or some days," 40 percent reported "most days," and 44 percent reported "every day."[22] In a similar study conducted with 5,014 adolescents between the ages of 12–15, 8.3 percent reported never having family dinner, 7.3 percent reported having family dinner 1–2 times per week, 13.4 percent reported a dinner rate of 3–4 times per week, 28.1 percent reported 5–6 times per week, and 42 percent reported every day.[23] If we define a high frequency of family meals as five or more meals per week, then based upon the studies quoted above, 45–70 percent of children in the United States report a high frequency of family meals. Whatever the reality, this large range shows that family meals are not consistent.

In the United States, most people who eat dinner with their families tend to eat breakfast alone and eat lunch with their classmates or coworkers.[24] So from

INDIVIDUALITY vs. COMMUNITY

the perspective of an American nuclear family for whom breakfast or lunch is not considered to have much of a familial context, the statistics on family meal

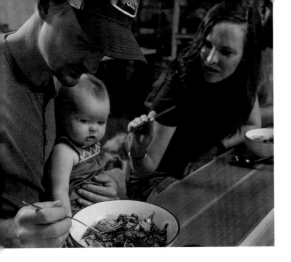

frequency may not seem that low or odd. But considering the 21 distinct meals we might eat in a week, the fact that potentially half of American children eat less than a quarter of those meals with their family is striking if not at least interesting. Writing about the demise of the family meal, Anne Murcott quotes an upset father who laments, "I ate only seven meals at home all last week and three of those were on Sunday."[25] While this father may not be happy about his situation, by a certain standard he's still considered to be on the high side of family meal frequency.

More alarming is the fact that these numbers seem to be improving in the wealthiest and most educated Americans but declining in the poorest and lowest educated. In a study conducted to assess trends in family meal frequency in the United States from 1999 to 2010, a high family meal frequency of five or more meals per week held relatively stable at 48.2 percent for a population of 3,072 kids surveyed in 1999 and 48.5 percent

for a population of 2,793 kids living in the same region who were surveyed in 2010. But when the data was analyzed based on socioeconomic status, the trend for high family meal frequency rose in the highest socioeconomic class from 55.8 percent in 1999 to 61.3 percent in 2010 and fell in the lowest socioeconomic class from 46.9 percent in 1999 to 38.8 percent in 2010. On average, kids from low socioeconomic backgrounds ate with their families 4 times per week in 1999 and 3.6 times per week in 2010. Besides declines in low socioeconomic classes, declines were also seen in girls, middle school students (grades 6–8), and Asians.[26]

Although the outlook for family meals in the United States isn't great (or is perhaps just inconsistent, especially in lower socioeconomic classes), the situation in the United Kingdom may be even worse. In one study assessing family meal frequency in Britain, only 33 percent of British youths reported a high frequency of family meals.[27]

The situation is quite different in other countries. In studies similar to the ones conducted on family meal frequency in the United States and Britain, 78 percent of Spanish youths report high rates of family meal frequency.[28] Likewise, in Canadian provinces such as Ontario and Nova Scotia, 70 percent of youths report a high frequency of family meals.[29]

But it's the French who seem to be excelling as a nation when it comes to creating consistent and structured meal

Though many of us intuitively feel that family meals are beneficial, there is also clear scientific evidence that children who eat more frequently with their families are physically and psychologically better off.

patterns for their children. In one study conducted by F. Bellisle and M. F. Rolland-Cachera, samples of 1,000 French children ages 9–11 were studied using standardized questionnaires to assess trends in physical activity, diet, and dietary habits over three distinct time periods (1993, 1995, and 1997). Over each of these three time periods, a strong and persistent meal structure was found. Almost all of the children ate breakfast (97 percent). All children had lunch (100 percent), with most (67 percent) having lunch at home and the rest (33 percent) in their school cafeteria. A traditional afternoon snack after school was consumed by the majority of children (88 percent). Finally, nearly all children (99 percent) had dinner, almost always at home with all family members (87 percent). Despite the fact that these children reported strong preferences for foods rich in sugar and fat, no abnormal data was reported for body mass index in children over the three distinct measure-ment times. If anything, there was a trend from 1993 to 1997 toward less television-watching, more physical activity, and a more complete breakfast.[30]

Compared to data from the United States, the French statistics are utopian, especially if we believe that family meals are important to our children's health and well-being. Though many of us intuitively feel that family meals are beneficial, there is also clear scientific evidence that children who eat more frequently with their families are physically and psychologically better off.[31]

First and foremost, family meals improve the diet quality and long-term eating habits of children.[32] Specifically, kids who eat more frequently with their families gravitate toward healthier foods such as fruits and vegetables and tend to stay away from unhealthy foods such as soft drinks and fast food. As a result, their intake of fiber is higher, as is their intake of important vitamins and minerals.[33] It's an effect that seems to last well into adulthood, as kids who eat more frequently with their families end up continuing their healthy food choices and eating habits, including cooking at home and eating with others as adults.[34] Of note, children who eat the same foods as their parents also have better diets and enjoy their food more. Based on this fact, parents don't need to give in to the pressure to let picky children demand a separate meal or dictate the entire meal.[35]

Beyond improving diet, higher family meal frequency may also stem obesity patterns in children. Some data shows that the odds of being obese are greater in kids who eat less frequently with their families.[36] But for kids who aren't already overweight or obese, the chances of becoming obese don't seem to be related to family meal frequency.[37] This relationship, however, may be specific to white children, who show lower odds of being obese with an

HEALTHY DIETS
HEALTHY vs. BEHAVIORS

increase in meal frequency, whereas black or Hispanic children do not seem to incur a protective effect from an increase in family meal frequency.[38] Finally, there is also data that does not describe a relationship between weight and family meal frequency, highlighting the fact that childhood obesity is a complex multifactorial problem but not diminishing the idea that family meals can be an important part of the overall solution.[39]

The most striking benefit of family meals, however, is not just physical —

it's psychological. Kids who eat more frequently with their families have lower rates of eating disorders such as binge eating, purging, or anorexia.[40] They exhibit less high-risk behavior, including substance abuse, violent acts, sexual promiscuity, and disciplinary problems at school.[41] High family meal frequency is also related to improved self-esteem and academic performance.[42] Frequent family meals are also associated with lower rates of depression and suicidal thoughts. Interestingly, the positive effect of family meals seems to be greater in girls than in boys, especially for factors such as disordered eating.[43]

Much of this psychosocial benefit may be explained by the simple fact that family meals improve communication between parents and their children.[44] Essentially, family meals give parents an opportunity to actually parent. In fact, it is thought that eating with our children is the basis for how we teach them basic social skills, ethics, language, and culture. For example, at only 12 months of age, young babies point at objects at the dinner table, not only because they want something but also because they want to share an experience. Not only do babies want to share food, they want to share emotions and a sense of belonging. From the very start of human life, eating together is essential to figuring out our basic relationship to others and the world.[45]

DIET-HEALTH PARADOX

Though it's hard to argue against the benefits of family meals for children, how this relates to public health is another question. Some insight can be drawn at the opposite end of the developmental spectrum by examining some of the paradoxical metrics surrounding the single largest killer in developed countries—cardiovascular disease and its manifestation as heart attacks and strokes.[46]

There are many risk factors for cardiovascular disease. They include physical inactivity, diabetes, smoking, obesity, hypertension, family history, and a high-fat diet.[47] For the most part, these risk factors are extremely robust and predictive, especially a diet high in saturated fats and cholesterol.[48] So much so that the American Heart Association and others recommend consuming a diet with less than 20 percent fat, with no more than 10 percent coming from saturated fat.[49]

However, for the French, these recommendations don't seem to apply. The "French paradox" is the observation that the French have extremely low rates of cardiovascular disease despite a high intake of dietary cholesterol and fat. There are reports that place the total fat consumption of the French in the range of 38–40 percent of total caloric intake, with saturated fat in the realm of 15 percent.[50]

Despite this high fat consumption, the World Health Organization reports that

from 2000 to 2007, the average age-standardized mortality rate in France from heart disease was 8.3 per 100,000. This is second only to Japan, which had a mortality rate from heart disease of 6.4 per 100,000 from 2000 to 2009. In contrast, from 2000 to 2005, the United States had a mortality rate from heart disease of 26.4 per 100,000—a death rate more than three times higher than the French and four times higher than the Japanese.[51]

This paradox doesn't exist only in France. This same pattern has also been observed and reported in the Catalunya region of Girona, Spain, the epicenter for English-speaking professional cyclists. Catalunya also exhibits a high cluster of cardiovascular risk factors but has lower rates of heart attacks than the rest of Spain, which already has the fourth lowest mortality from heart disease in the developed world at 11.7 per 100,000 from 2000 to 2008.[52]

There are many explanations for the French paradox, in both France and other regions exhibiting this phenomenon. These explanations include the possibility of underreporting deaths related to cardiovascular disease, a higher polyphenol intake from red wine, which may be protective to the heart, a higher consumption of fruits and vegetables, more consistent physical activity (i.e., not sitting all day), and a more holistic attitude about food that emphasizes higher quality, more diverse foods, and sharing meals.[53]

The differences in our cultural attitudes about food play a more important role in this health disparity because they directly shape *how we eat.*

Although all of these factors are important and likely play a role in explaining the French paradox, it's cultural differences in our attitudes about food and its role in community that I find most interesting.

Compared to the French and other cultures that demonstrate a diet-health paradox, Americans emphasize quantity over quality. We like things that make life easier, comforts and convenience, over things that make life interesting, experiences and joy. We revel in abundance while the French prefer moderation. We're a nation of large menus and highly

individual rather than communal notions of food.

When Americans are asked about food, they deconstruct their diets, discussing elements of food such as carbohydrate, fat, or protein. They don't simply talk in terms of identifiable foods. Americans also personalize their food, identifying themselves with a type of diet such as vegan, Paleo, Mediterranean, vegetarian, clean-eating, dairy-free, organic, gluten-free, non-GMO, or low-carb. In the United States, food is seen as the responsibility of the individual, with personal health cited as the top reason for one's diet choices. Ironically, as a nation, those "healthy" diets don't seem to be working.

However, when the French are asked about food, they talk about actual foods such as bread, cheese, and the vegetables growing in their garden. They talk about the quality and freshness of those whole-food ingredients and share recipes. Discussions about food are not individualized. Ideas about what to eat are based on one's relationship with others. It's not just about what's being served, it's about who's coming over for dinner. Taste matters more than health, which means that sugar and fat are used in relatively greater amounts. Rarely does a French person discuss his or her dietary restrictions or the health and performance goals that individual diets are designed for.[54]

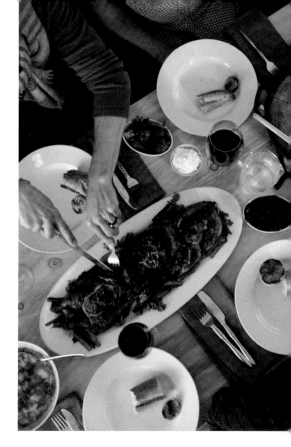

Because differences in cardiovascular disease between the French and Americans aren't explained by *what we eat*, especially with respect to total fat and saturated fat, it's likely that the differences in our cultural attitudes about food play a more important role in this health disparity because they directly shape *how we eat*.

If there's one single or culminating behavior that best explains the French paradox, it's simply that the French eat less than Americans do. In French restaurants, portion sizes are smaller, as are individually wrapped portions of food in French supermarkets. Even French cookbooks list a higher serving number for a given amount of food. Of note, not only do the French eat less than Americans do, they also take much longer to eat, relishing in the experience rather than just trying to get on with their day.[55] How is it that the French eat less but take longer to eat? The simple answer is that they eat together.[56]

In fact, as studies on French and American family meal frequency and structure clearly demonstrate, the French eat together in orders of magnitude more than Americans do. I can't help but think that this is a critical though rarely discussed explanation for why Americans die from heart attacks at a rate three times higher than the French. Rarely does someone just linger over a small meal by themselves.

Given the countless factors that are responsible for cardiovascular disease,

it may seem far-fetched that one behavior—eating together—may be a key to preventing cardiovascular disease. Certainly the people we eat with can reinforce both negative and positive behaviors.[57] So just coming together isn't enough. Still, France isn't the only place in the world where the combination of eating with family and a positive social dynamic is linked with a diet-health paradox.

In Japan, fast-food restaurants such as McDonald's and Kentucky Fried Chicken, as well as indigenous fast-food restaurants including ramen shops and sushi bars that dispense food on conveyer belts, are extremely popular. They have become a normal part of the Japanese landscape, especially in busy, densely packed cities.[58]

Like many, I think of fast-food restaurants as the epitome of unhealthy eating, responsible for a variety of health problems including obesity, type 2 diabetes, and cardiovascular disease.[59] Fast-food restaurants and chains are also symbolic of the social woe and blight of modern American urban sprawl. Their convenience and low prices, as well as their ubiquity in poor neighborhoods, create "food deserts" where healthy foods are no longer available. Access to local, organic, or whole foods has become a class-defining resource, inequitably allocated to wealthy neighborhoods.[60] In the United States, fast-food restaurants represent an anomie,

FAMILY-STYLE
FOR ALL TO SHARE

a situation where society provides little moral guidance to individuals because of a breakdown between the social bonds linking individuals with their community.[61]

But in Japan, the nation with the lowest rate of cardiovascular disease in the developed world, fast-food restaurants are not the urban anomie they are in the United States. Rather, they are locations where families and friends across generations share food in an intimate and convivial manner. Instead of eating fast food alone, which is common in the United States, most Japanese dine together. And instead of ordering individually, they order multiple items on the menu and consume their food "family-style," taking bites of the same burger or fish sandwich, laying out one order of french fries in the center of the table for all to share, and purchasing only one or two sodas, then sharing the same straw. Despite being a nontraditional type of food and food system, the convenience and mechanization of fast food in Japan has not changed traditional social dynamics or patterns of eating together.[62]

Diets high in saturated fats are clearly associated with higher rates of cardiovascular disease, as is eating out frequently. That said, what diet-health paradoxes in places like France and Japan demonstrate is that it's not solely about what one eats when it comes to a society's health. It's also about how we eat and who we eat with—that we need both people and food to be fully satiated.

LONELINESS

It's been over 20 years since I've been to a McDonald's in the United States. But as much as I despise McDonald's, when I first moved to Girona, Spain, it was one of my guilty pleasures. Although working on the Pro Cycling Tour was a dream come true, I was at times deeply lonely.

I would get off the plane in Barcelona feeling jet-lagged, alone, and tired—and if the temperature was a little too hot across the jet bridge or if the smell of floor cleaner that they used to polish the linoleum was too strong, I'd have a mini-panic attack. I called it "crumple vibes"—an intensely claustrophobic feeling, like I was trapped in a tight aluminum can that was on the verge of being crushed. To cope, I'd take a few deep breaths, tell myself that everything was going to be okay, and then think, *If my luggage comes out early, I can be in Girona in less than two hours and grab a Filet-O-Fish and fries.* That thought, that little mission, those fries and that sandwich relieved my anxiety and helped me deal with the fact that I was homesick.

The theory of social surrogacy posits that certain objects, scents, sounds—nonhuman stimuli—can create a sense of belonging because of prior emotional connections between that stimuli and the people who are important to us. Our need to be connected leads us to seek out nonhuman surrogates—for example, a familiar television show—when we feel lonely.[63] For better or worse, food is also a strong social surrogate, because many of the foods we eat are intimately connected with our friends and family. In a study on the effect of comfort foods, Troisi and Gabriel found that these foods activated relationship-related connections and that the degree to which a food sparked these connections matched how comforting a person thought that food was. For example, while many of us might feel that chicken noodle soup is a comfort food, if someone doesn't have an association between chicken noodle soup and an important relationship, then that person won't consider chicken noodle soup to be comforting. Troisi and Gabriel also found that like other social surrogates, comfort foods are a powerful buffer against loneliness.[64]

Living in Europe was its own sort of immigration for me and the many American cyclists I coached. The experience was reminiscent of when my family first

There's a thin line between game-day swagger and the actual bottleneck of depression and emotional turbulence that we are all susceptible to, whether from the monotony and effort of daily training far from home or the basic rigors of life.

immigrated to the United States. When I was a little kid, my dad would take my older brother and me to McDonald's on the days that my mom was in school or working. We would get so excited to go. For us, eating at McDonald's was a privilege and a treat. What I inadvertently discovered when I started working in Europe was that McDonald's was comfort food for me in those moments of intense loneliness.

The loneliness I experienced is rarely, if ever, discussed in professional sports. But I think it's more common than people let on. After his horrific crash at the national championships in 2014, Taylor Phinney, one of America's preeminent professional cyclists with two Olympic berths and multiple world championship titles, found himself back home in Boulder, Colorado. Despite his grave injuries, the terrible upset of being sidelined from racing, and the temporary loss of his basic mobility, the silver lining was having time to reconnect with old friends. It was a glimpse of the life that he gave up to live and race in Europe.

When Taylor first turned professional, he moved to the Tuscany region of Italy and then later to Nice, France. Having spent his early childhood in Italy, Taylor was already fluent in Italian and took pride in assimilating to European life with more ease than many of his peers. What he discovered in reuniting with his friends and family was that his bravado about living on his own was a mask that disguised periods of intense loneliness. Although the majority of English-speaking riders live in Girona, Spain, Taylor has always been reticent to live there, in part because he saw the concentration of American riders as a crutch. So I was a bit surprised when he told me that when he returned to racing in Europe, he planned to be based in Girona. When I asked him why he was going to move again, he was frank: "When I'm in Nice, I've got no one to eat with."

As much as athletes talk about having their head in the game or being tough, performance isn't just about having the willpower or talent to suffer on the field. There's a thin line between game-day swagger and the actual bottleneck of depression and emotional turbulence that we are all susceptible to, whether from the monotony and effort of daily training far from home or the basic rigors of life. In my own time spent coaching athletes in

Europe, I discovered firsthand that nothing could bolster or rate-limit performance as much as one's mental well-being. A simple dinner with great company could inspire the power to win, while something as seemingly benign and common as loneliness could be the loose thread that, when pulled, unraveled everything. Whether I was feeling lonely or the athletes I coached were, our physical or mental work performance was hampered.

One of the innate problems of being an athlete (or just driven), however, is the incessant pursuit to be better, which means the thread is being tugged all the time. In his book *Loneliness*, Dr. Clark Moustakas defines loneliness anxiety as "a fundamental breach between what one is and what one pretends to be."[65] Athletes are always imagining and dreaming. Caught in possibility, the best are constantly working to take their game to the next level so they can be more than they already are. As much as we revere this ambition, the downside is that athletes risk becoming disconnected from who they actually are when they are chasing a future version of themselves, especially when that version is being constantly showcased and praised by social media. The elation of victory can easily turn to dread, as athletes must repeatedly produce results to prove their value once again. Likewise, failing in the midst of strong personal and public expectation can turn ugly if not framed as external to one's identity. There's a big difference between a person saying "I failed" and "I'm a failure."

In trying to understand my anecdotal observation that loneliness can physically hurt athletic capacity, I discovered an extensive body of scientific literature on the opposite end of the performance spectrum demonstrating that loneliness, isolation, and a lack of social support can literally make us sick and prematurely kill us. None of us would doubt that smoking a cigarette before running a mile all-out will hamper our speed. But we might pause at the suggestion by Dr. Guy Winch that loneliness is as much of a threat to our physical health as cigarettes—an idea we remain ignorant to because, as Winch puts

PHYSICAL vs. **NEEDS** **EMOTIONAL** **NEEDS**

it, "Cigarettes come with a warning label; loneliness does not."[66]

Winch isn't wrong in his assessment. A lack of social connection and loneliness

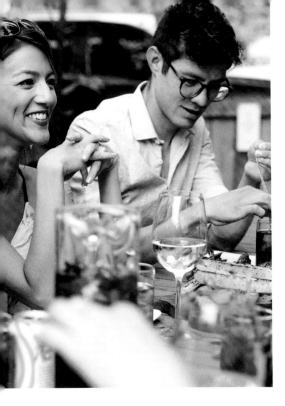

body mass index—found that loneliness was independently related to cardiovascular disease in women but not men.[69] This difference may be explained by reports that women tend to be affected more adversely by loneliness than men, as well as reports that men typically report much higher rates of isolation and loneliness than women.[70] So it's possible that while loneliness affects the health of women more negatively, more men are lonely, creating a data set that may bias toward one gender, depending upon how the data is gathered. That said, what is clear is that data linking loneliness with cardiovascular disease exists for both genders.

Loneliness is as detrimental to our physical and mental health as any major health epidemic or risk factor.

is bad for our hearts, increasing the risk for heart disease and the inflammation that may be directly related to blood vessel damage just like the damage done by cigarettes.[67]

In one particular study, this increase in heart disease risk from loneliness was also linked to a higher resting heart rate—an independent risk factor by itself—with loneliness affecting those in lower socioeconomic classes more, especially men.[68] In contrast, a different study—after controlling for depressive symptoms, age, race, education, income, marital status, hypertension, diabetes, cholesterol, physical activity, smoking, alcohol use, systolic and diastolic blood pressure, and

Not only does loneliness spawn cardiovascular problems, but also when patients are already sick, those who are lonely do worse compared to others with the same level of illness, requiring more days in the hospital and more readmissions to the hospital.[71] Whether it's a cold or a chronic disease, those who are lonely use the emergency room more and incur more medical costs than those who are not lonely.[72] This seems to also mirror the observation that athletes perceive their

It's clear that eating together is independently related to improved health and happiness and needs to be recognized as an important strategy for buffering loneliness.

injuries to be worse than they actually are when they are lonely.[73]

Loneliness and social isolation in the elderly are also independently linked to higher rates of diabetes, hypertension, liver disease, arthritis, emphysema, tuberculosis, kidney disease, asthma, and stroke across ethnic groups.[74] The net effect is that loneliness increases one's risk for death. Of particular concern is the fact that increases in premature mortality associated with loneliness don't just occur in people who are chronically lonely; relatively recent changes in feelings of loneliness can also increase risk of mortality, demonstrating that the negative effects on our health may be both chronic and acute.[75]

There may be a direct biological mechanism responsible for this increase in mortality. As cells replicate, the DNA in our chromosomes, which contain all of the code that makes us who we are, is also copied. The tips of our chromosomes are protected by noncoding caps called telomeres. As cells go through more cell divisions and get older, the telomeres shorten, and this shortening is thought to be directly related to aging, mortality, and age-related diseases.[76] What's incredible is that low social support in older individuals

(65–84 years) is associated with shorter telomere length compared to the same age range of individuals with high social support, regardless of ethnicity or gender.[77] This fascinating research effectively shows that loneliness causes us to age faster on a cellular and genetic level, especially toward the latter part of life.

Furthermore, loneliness and isolation have been shown to reduce cognitive function in the elderly—verbal fluency, immediate recall, and delayed recall.[78] Loneliness also directly predicts unhealthy dietary habits and malnutrition in older adults. Eating alone and loneliness in elderly people is a predictor of both anorexia and obesity.[79] This nutritional risk can be offset by home meal delivery services, in part because having someone stop by to deliver food also serves to decrease loneliness and increase social interaction.[80]

In fact, loneliness is associated with a wide spectrum of disordered eating across all ages, from anorexia and bulimia to binge eating and obesity.[81] This association between disordered eating and loneliness parallels the observation that elite athletes have a much higher rate of eating disorders than the general population.[82] Although disordered eating in athletes is thought to be directly related to making weight for performance reasons, I can't help but hypothesize that whether causative or not, the severity of disordered eating in athletes is also related to the degree of loneliness they experience.[83]

Given how closely linked loneliness is to so many different health and behavioral problems, instead of treating those problems on their own or seeing them as singular issues, alleviating the root cause of someone's loneliness needs to be part of the remedy for an illness or performance decline that exists in conjunction with loneliness. Unfortunately, as common as loneliness may be to the human condition, it's the very ubiquity of loneliness across a diverse spectrum of people that also makes it a complex, multifaceted, and highly individual experience with innumerable causes and consequences.[84] A single panacea is unlikely.

This complexity, however, doesn't discount the specific relationship between eating alone and loneliness as a crucial piece to this very intricate puzzle. In one of the largest studies of its kind, an eight-year national study on happiness was conducted in Thailand to track the lives of 39,820 individuals from 2005 to 2013 in order to better understand the connection between happiness and health. Data from 2009 to 2013 showed that eating alone was significantly related to being unhappy, lonely, and sick. And though older single men were the ones who were most likely to eat alone, women suffered more unhappiness from eating by themselves than men did.[85] Based on this and similar studies, it's clear that eating together is independently related to improved health and happiness and needs to be recognized as an important strategy for buffering loneliness.[86]

Not only does eating together improve happiness and health, the act of eating together also holds us accountable. That is, those who tend to eat more when they are alone eat less when they are with others, and those who don't tend to eat enough when alone eat more when with others.[87] In one study, researchers found that people who feel socially disconnected eat about twice as much as those who feel connected or included.[88] The bottom line is that as much as loneliness and eating alone can hurt how and what we eat, eating together can help reverse those issues.

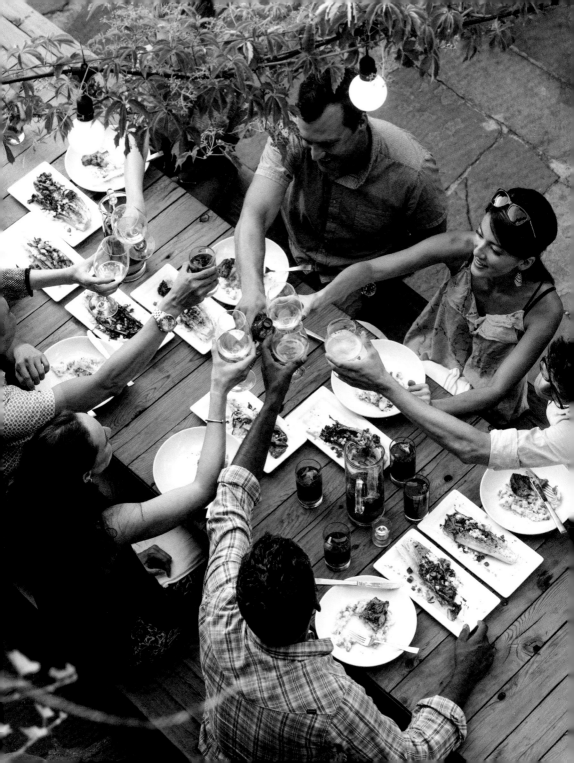

"WE" VERSUS "I"

All told, we are complicated people with very simple needs—food and belonging being two of the most important. Insomuch as the roots of loneliness are multifactorial, with both internal and external facets, so are the barriers that keep us from eating together.

While some of the barriers aren't surmountable—for example, the passing of a loved one—in many cases they are. Reaching out to old friends, extending oneself to make new ones, or taking the time to learn to cook might be obstacles that when solved not only bring people to the table but also address loneliness beyond the context of food.[89] Not only is the act of eating together a direct solution for loneliness, solving the problems that keep us from eating together may be as well.

To be clear, being alone, by itself, is not a cause of loneliness. If anything, alone time can actually be a precious source of renewal for many in this busy world.[90] But whether we are choosing to cherish time by ourselves or stubbornly suffering in our own isolation, it's important to realize that what we do or don't do to take care of ourselves has consequences, not just for us as individuals but also for everyone close to us. Whether good or bad, our physical and mental health is literally contagious.[91]

We might think that only viruses are infectious, but loneliness can spread between people within a social network like a contagion. If you are lonely, it's very likely that your friends are lonely too, spreading up to three degrees of separation. Loneliness is very much a cause and consequence of becoming disconnected. And once one becomes disconnected, the dominoes just keep falling as the lonely get pushed out farther to the periphery by a group, consciously or unconsciously, protecting themselves from becoming infected.[92] This social contagion phenomenon has also been observed for depression, smoking, divorce, alcohol consumption, obesity, dietary patterns and heart disease, and health traits such as body mass index and blood pressure.[93] Essentially, whether you're sick or healthy, those close to you are probably the same. With this in mind, we may not only be what we eat. For better or for worse, we may also be who we eat with.

The situation, however, is not hopeless. In the same way that negative physical and mental health outcomes can spread, happiness is also infectious. As part of the Framingham Heart Study, 4,739 individuals were evaluated over a 20-year period, from 1983 to 2003. It was found that happiness, like loneliness and lifestyle-related diseases, can extend up to three degrees of separation. People who are surrounded by happy people and also active in their network are more likely to be happy in the future. In fact, if you aren't happy but become happy, there is a one in four chance that you will infect someone within a mile of you with that same happiness. This happiness effect, just like other infections, decays with time and geographical distance. Happiness spreads between spouses, siblings, family members, friends, and neighbors, but, interestingly, does not appear to spread between coworkers. It seems professional goals are not stronger than personal bonds. Ultimately, our happiness depends very much on the happiness of those closest to us, not just those working around us.[94]

Eventually, as the American athletes I coached began assimilating to European culture and started making friends outside of our team, we all suffered less loneliness and became stronger, happier, and better. Over time, we realized that our bottleneck wasn't talent or motivation. We began to learn basic life skills that allowed us to take better care of ourselves and each other. Fortunately, we acquired many of those life skills by being open to the incredible food and people in the Girona region of Catalunya. Though at

first foreign to us, Girona has a vibrant, age-old food culture similar to France and the rest of the Mediterranean. We discovered the local markets, taught ourselves how to cook, and as we became more versed in the slow-food culture of our adopted home, we became more comfortable integrating our newfound knowledge with our own American tastes.

In my case, that manifested in a greater interest in re-creating the simple Chinese dishes that I grew up with, which not only decreased my rogue trips to McDonald's but brought truly distinct recipes, such as portable rice cakes, to the European peloton. Although we were far from home and not always immune to loneliness, we were lucky to be part of a phenomenal team and to live in an incredible community that allowed us to be our quirky selves when we

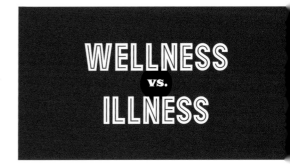

gathered around tables full of beautiful food. As Dr. Dean Ornish so profoundly puts it, the only difference between wellness and illness is "we" versus "I."[95]

CULTURAL DILEMMA

There may be a scientific basis for the perfect diet, whether for health or athletic performance, but given how differently some cyclists eat from one another and how similar those same cyclists perform, I've come to realize that the human body is extraordinarily adaptable, so physiology alone doesn't offer us a clear approach to food.

Further complicating the matter, as Americans, our food culture has steadily shifted from one that we predominately inherited from our families (ethnocentric) to one that is now more driven by technology (technocentric).[96] These lifestyles encompass a wide spectrum, from those that are still entirely rooted in tradition to those that are primarily driven by innovation. At one extreme, for example, we have Amish communities in the United States that eschew technology, growing and eating their food in exactly the same way as the generations who came before them did. At the other extreme, we have Silicon Valley "life hackers" who drink engineered meals so they can have more time to code software that is labeled according to its version number, just like the fuel they consume.[97] While most of us fall somewhere closer to the middle of the spectrum, it's clear that as we continue to modernize, new technologies play a bigger role in our everyday lives to the extent that much of our evolving culture is dictated to us by innovation and the unlikely pairing of science and consumerism that feeds it.

Ironically, we've come to embrace this shift toward progress and technology as part of our own tradition or culture. If anything, we inherit possibility and instability—both the gratification that comes from reinventing ourselves if we're not happy and the anguish of constantly reinventing ourselves to stay happy as progress creates unforeseen change. Richard Eckersley, who studies in detail how specific cultural factors such as materialism and individualism affect public health, calls the promotion of rapid progress and the images and ideals of "the good life" associated with independence and consumerism a cultural fraud because they directly impair our psychological and physical health rather than benefit them.[98]

Known as relative deprivation, the basic phenomenon is that even when all of our basic needs are met and we are otherwise healthy, if we feel that we are deprived relative to others we can exhibit psychosomatic disorders—actual physical illness—resulting from our sense of psychological or social deprivation.[99] Pharmaceutical companies have taken advantage of a variant of this phenomenon, increasing the market for specific drugs by convincing otherwise healthy populations through targeted advertising that they are suffering from the signs and symptoms treated only by those drugs—a tactic known as disease mongering.[100] It's a false reality that creates very real consequences that are perpetuated and reinforced by a media complex that is quick to cry wolf.[101]

Whether it's an illness we don't have or a thing we don't need, the incessant marketing of products and lifestyles in Western culture makes it difficult for most not to feel some sense of relative deprivation. Ironically, as we slay ourselves in "keeping up with the Joneses," driven by our strong desire for independence, we suffer even more when we fail to be a part of the group. In medicine and athletics, this failure to meet expectations and the resulting woe are also referred to as the "nocebo effect"—sickness or drops in performance stemming from the belief that one does not have the same medicine or technological advantages as others.[102]

For me, this cultural dilemma reached a tipping point at the pinnacle of my career, when I was hired to oversee the sport science program for Lance Armstrong and the RadioShack cycling team during what would be Armstrong's final professional season. For all of his achievements and his failings, no one I knew embodied the drive for innovation and success or the conflict between fame and loneliness more than Armstrong. Regardless of how people view him today, his rise and fall is very much an American story.

Ironically, as we slay ourselves in "keeping up with the Joneses," driven by our strong desire for independence, we suffer even more when we fail to be a part of the group.

When it came to the cutting edge, Armstrong was exceptionally motivated, curious, and willing to experiment. As a sport scientist, working with Armstrong was incredible. He was generous, methodical, and extraordinarily self-aware when it came to his physical performance. While he openly engaged all of my questions and ideas regarding his form, equipment, nutrition, training, and tactics, the one thing he would never entertain were the zany Kokology games I loved to play. Originally developed by Japanese psychologists Tadahiko Nagao and Isamu Saito, Kokology is designed to probe one's psyche with imaginary scenarios and questions to reveal hidden feelings. For fun, I'd lay out a scene for Armstrong, saying to him, "Imagine you're riding a camel across an endless desert and after days without food and almost no water you finally reach an oasis." Then I'd spring on him the question "Who's at the oasis?" His answer for any of these games or questions was always the same—a firm headshake and a definitive "No, Al, no," to which I would burst out laughing. I could never get him to answer.

I don't think even the most scientific and neurotic athletes I know choose to eat alone because they've been able to prove that doing so is better for their performance.

But when it came to going faster, he was always game. From field tests we knew that he was more aerodynamic on his time trial bicycle if he kept his head down. While great for aerodynamics, it's bad for seeing the road ahead. One day, I mused to Armstrong that it would be great if we could somehow use his iPhone so he wouldn't have to lift his head to see where he was going. The next thing I heard was, "Hey, Steve, how are you? . . . I've got a project I need some help with." Without hesitation he had called Steve Jobs to see if Apple could help build a phone for us that could be used as both a periscope and a cycling computer. Within a few days, my friend Michael Tseng was on the phone with Apple engineers, and within a week or so he had an iPhone jerry-rigged with mirrors and an app that corrected the onscreen image, ready for us to test before we moved forward. Excited, we mounted the phone between the time trial bars and Armstrong started pedaling with his head down. After less than a mile, he stopped. He said he couldn't ride with it—that seeing the shaking road ahead through the screen gave him vertigo. Although the idea didn't pan out, the fact that he could manifest a spitballing conversation into an actual proof of concept and have an answer in under two weeks was unreal.

From the perspective of technology and innovation, no one could compete with Armstrong's will, acumen, and resources. His celebrity, however, made it extremely difficult for him to function as an everyday person. If we were on the road and needed to stop for food or coffee, he would stay in the car as I went into the store or café to place the order. But the team dinners and meals at races were the most difficult things to manage. Because of the attention Armstrong would get wherever we went, it was extremely hard to have him at the dinner table with his teammates without attracting fans, journalists, sponsors, and looky-loos who distracted everyone at the table. We needed private dining rooms and extra security at events. By the time we were at the Tour de France, it was often easier for Armstrong to have his meals in his hotel room by himself. Despite our access to science and technology, we couldn't fix the fact that because of his fame, Armstrong was often isolated from his own team. Looking back at it, my feeling is that all of the factors playing into that single circumstance negated much of what we tried to do scientifically to improve his performance. Like glacier melt, not being able to eat together was a sign of a bigger crisis.

In a certain way, Armstrong's experience personifies a challenge we all face in modern America. Our desire to be independent and successful puts ever-increasing demands on us and on our time. This can keep us from connecting with our kids, parents, friends, partners, and teammates over what used to be the most common and familial activity—eating. And when we become disconnected, it sets up a cycle of isolation and loneliness, which drives us to feel we need more money or possessions so we can distract ourselves from discomfort with novelty instead of reality. Every day I see people staring into their smartphones in need of connection, and it reminds me of how I used to stare out the window as a latchkey kid waiting for my mom and dad to come home from work. It's the same thing. In a technocentric culture, we're all latchkey kids. Unfortunately, rather than helping us

with our loneliness, technology just seems to be making us better at being together yet still alone.[103]

By the very nature of competition, this cultural dilemma is at the heart of sports. The Olympic motto, *Citius, Altius, Fortius*, or "faster, higher, stronger," captures values and a mind-set innate to both athletics and a technocentric society. For most athletes, if the major downside of going faster, reaching higher, and being stronger is eating

TECHNOLOGY vs. CULTURE

alone, then most will gladly do so. Still, I don't think even the most scientific and neurotic athletes I know choose to eat alone because they've been able to prove that doing so is better for their performance. Even the best athletes in the world are susceptible to the same cultural and life stressors placed on all of us in our modern world. So while athletes may have the added pressure of needing to be more careful about their diet for performance reasons, it doesn't remove the external burdens that might be hampering the time or skills they need to prepare great meals for themselves or others. Because of these burdens, eating alone might make attending to one's nutrition more convenient and even less stressful, but that doesn't mean it's actually the better way to eat for performance. And though the argument can be made that beyond my anecdotal observations there's no direct evidence that eating alone specifically hurts athletic performance, there's certainly clear evidence that eating alone hurts people. Ultimately, I come from the perspective that all athletes are human, even if not all humans consider themselves athletes.

That said, if the issue is solely about reaching the pinnacle of performance and if winning the Tour de France is used as the measuring stick, then I concede that my ideas about a cultural dilemma and performance are wrong. Over the past 20 years the majority of Tour de France winners have not come from ethnocentric, family meal–eating cultures. They've come from highly technical and scientific-based programs. From the disgraced Americans to the most recent dominance by Britain's Team Sky, it's clear that being technocentric creates winners. In fact, not since Bernard Hinault won his last Tour de France in 1985 has a French rider won the Tour de France. The French may not be winning their own national race, but who's to say that they aren't winning at life?

After British rider Bradley Wiggins won the Tour de France in 2012, he announced that he would not be coming back to defend his title despite still being in his prime. Having worked with Wiggins in the past, I couldn't help but assume that after experiencing the physical and psychological rigors of winning the Tour de France, he realized that winning just wasn't worth the cost. I also couldn't help but wonder what might have happened if he were allowed to take a more humanistic approach to his preparation. Perhaps he knows it wouldn't have been possible to win that way. Or perhaps he would still have the motivation and capacity to win more Tours. Regardless, I found Wiggins's decision not to defend his title incredibly thought-provoking and inspiring.

So what's the solution? Do we choose to be winners or do we choose to be happy? My sense is that we can have our cake and eat it too. We don't have to put down our modern conveniences and regress to an agrarian lifestyle, nor do we have to turn into soulless robots connected to each other by Wi-Fi. The bright side of innovation and progress is that it is innately optimistic. Learning and greatness occur when we struggle, practice, and push beyond our boundaries until we fail.[104] Rather than see as a problem the stress we put on ourselves and the many inevitable mistakes that occur when we do, the talented see stress as an opportunity to learn and correct—to be open to both new scientific fact and timeless traditions. It's the only way we find the sweet spot.

NUTRITIONAL PRAGMATISM

Over the course of my career as a sport scientist, I fully embraced and cultivated a technocentric lifestyle and the highly individualistic and reductionist view of nutrition I was taught in school. This is a total contrast to the ethnocentric and communal perspective of food that I later discovered as key to maintaining connection and resilience in both sport and life.

As a scientist, I think about nutrition in terms of the total calories, carbohydrate, water, and sodium a specific person needs for his or her individual goals. I wonder about the antioxidants and phytochemicals in an apple rather than the wide variety of apples that I've been told used to grow in my neighborhood. But as a human being, I want to belong and share the beautiful sight, smell, and taste of a home-cooked meal with my family and friends. I want to peruse my local farmers' market and learn timeless recipes to nurture myself and others. My personal experience and the advice I give to those trying to balance these two sides—the technocentric and ethnocentric—is to practice nutritional pragmatism rather than nutritional extremism.

When I finished my PhD in physiology, one thing I was certain of was that I had more questions than answers—that I didn't even know what I didn't know—that the human body, nature, and the universe are so vast, complex, and intricate that contra-diction is the norm, and that very little of the immense variability we see in biological data has yet to be explained by science.

One of my favorite studies reminds me of this fact. The study examined iron absorption in a group of Thai and Swed-ish women, following a previous study that found Thai women's iron absorption from a traditional meal to be lower than expected.[105] To better understand what might be hindering iron absorption in the Thai women, the follow-up study compared Thai women based in Thailand to Swedish women based in Sweden who were known to be normal. As a part of the control, the researchers fed both groups wheat rolls for-tified with the same amount of a traceable isotope of iron. Likewise, the researchers fed both groups a traditional Thai dish of rice, vegetables, and chili paste, which was also fortified with the same amount of traceable iron. The foods were prepared in the respective countries, then frozen and shipped to the women in the study. Of note, "the amount of chili paste was smaller" in the dishes shipped to Sweden because "the Swedish subjects had difficulties taking the same amount as the Thai subjects." When both groups were given the wheat rolls, there was a "higher average absorption from wheat observed in the Swedish women" compared to the Thai women. But when both groups were given the traditional Thai dish, "the Thai subjects absorbed more iron from the meals than the Swedish subjects." In the discussion, the authors stated, "The Swedish women liked the meal but considered it very spicy. It might be that the strong spices in some way interfered with the absorption of iron in the Swedish women (altered gastrointestinal motility, lowered secretion of gastric juices, etc.)."[106]

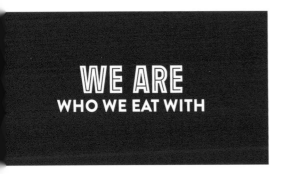

WE ARE
WHO WE EAT WITH

On one hand, these studies used a relatively brand-new technique at the time to study iron absorption, and the papers were chock-full of strange methodological problems and a results section that was very difficult to understand, especially with respect to what was actually happening with the wheat roll data between groups, all of which may have affected the results. On the other hand, maybe people just absorb more nutrients from the foods they are familiar with and like to eat. Maybe culture and taste matter. Either way, it's clear that there's more to nutrition than simply reducing food to little bits and pieces.

Likewise, optimal diets or ingredients must be considered in context. Recently, an article by Robert H. Lustig and others was published in *Nature* claiming that refined sugar is toxic and needs to be regulated like alcohol and tobacco.[107] The authors directly blame sugar consumption for increases in obesity, diabetes, and metabolic disorders. A separate paper responding to the *Nature* article lambasted Lustig and his colleagues for nutritional extremism, reminding readers that physical activity, one's overall diet, and total energy balance also play a critical role in obesity, diabetes, and other metabolic diseases and that a single ingredient cannot be blamed. Belkova and others ask, "Is the effort to 'outlaw' sugars a symptom of nutritional extremism that can be as harmful as any other type of extremism?"[108] Nutritional pragmatism put into practice suggests that any form of extremism is harmful — everything has to be evaluated with the big picture in mind, including what we eat. That's the nature of being pragmatic.

It's not about chastising a food as unhealthy, it's about promoting behaviors

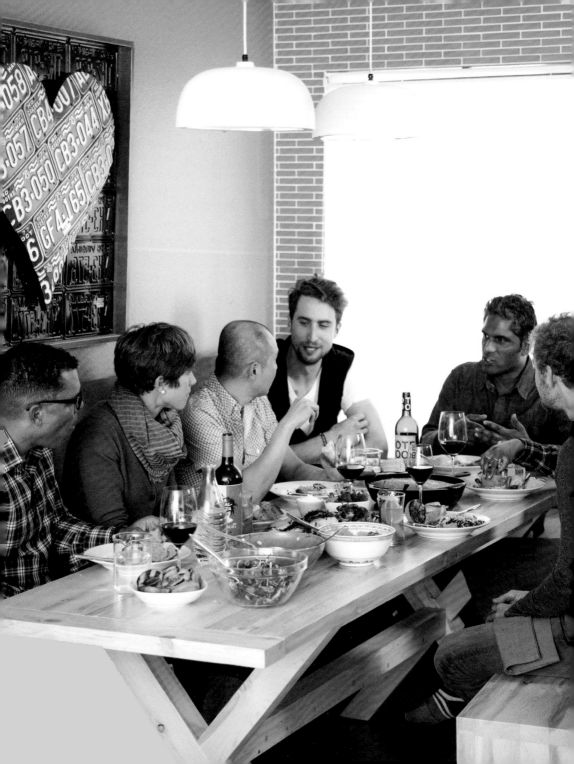

Nutritional pragmatism put into practice suggests that any form of extremism is harmful—everything has to be evaluated with the big picture in mind, including what we eat. That's the nature of being pragmatic.

around foods that are healthy. The bigger problem is not so much what to eat, it's about making the time to shop, cook a meal, and get everyone around the same table at the same time to eat it.

How do you do that? My simple answer is, I don't know. We all have very different life situations and problems that require their own unique solutions. I do know that if you want to make it happen, you will. There are creative answers out there.

When I was a kid, my parents worked incredibly hard to make ends meet. From bagging groceries at the local supermarket to a failed attempt at a Chinese restaurant, their life wasn't always easy. Eventually, my mom went back to school to become a pharmacist and my dad started a clothing business with one of my uncles. With two working parents, my brother and I were left unsupervised at home. But we weren't without responsibility. With so little time, my parents counted on me and my brother to help with the food prep before they came home from work. It was the only way they could pull off family dinners. So by the time we were in the third and fourth grades—just old enough to know how serious it was to use a knife—Mom began

giving us specific tasks to attend to when we got home from school. They included cutting and washing vegetables, rinsing and prepping rice, and making sure any frozen meat was thawed. Almost every afternoon we'd get a call from my mom, checking in to make sure we knew what we were doing. As soon as my parents came home, we'd start the rice cooker, and if everything was done right, the prepped vegetables and meat would be thrown in a wok and dinner would be ready as soon as the rice was done cooking. I know that from my parents' perspective, having us do food prep at such a young age wasn't ideal. We often complained about our chores, and I know that not being home with us weighed heavily on my parents. But their solution for maintaining a tradition of family meals was pragmatic, and it ended up giving us useful life skills. Most important, we always had dinner together.

Even today, I stress over putting meals together for myself and my friends. I remember one day last summer I was pretty proud of myself for taking the time to put a small roast in the oven in the morning to slow-cook all day. On a bike ride with Taylor Phinney, I invited him to stop by for dinner. By the time we rolled back into town it was about 7 p.m. Right before we parted ways he said, "How about 7:30? Can I bring a friend or two?" I yelled back, "Yeah, no problem." Arriving home, I quickly changed clothes and pulled the small roast out of the oven—it tasted amazing. I was pretty stoked.

Eventually Taylor showed up with an entourage. Eight additional people had either heard about my roast from Taylor or smelled my roast and showed up to check it out. I scrambled to prepare more rice, put some extra meat on the grill, and start making more salad as quickly as possible. I was in the weeds, hustling and directing my guests and working as hard as possible to feed everyone who just showed up. I got the service done, bellies were filled, and everyone seemed happy. As people started leaving, Taylor stayed behind to talk. His words caught me totally off guard. First, he thanked me for dinner and apologized for showing up with so many unexpected guests. Then he took me out to the woodshed, criticizing me for being so stressed out and not present at the meal

and with the company. At first, I wanted to disagree with him, but he was right. I was too concerned about feeding everyone to actually enjoy myself or be social. As he said goodbye, Taylor said, "Your food's great, man, but nobody really cares. We just want to hang out."

Make the time to shop, cook a meal, and get everyone around the table at the same time to eat it.

Since that day, I don't make a big deal out of having people over for food. Instead of worrying about having dishes ready at a specific time or pretending that it took no work to pull off a meal, I invite people over to hang out while I cook. Instead of choosing extravagant recipes to impress others, I cook what I would make if I were eating by myself—like a simple omelet over sushi rice. The bottom line is that things don't have to be fancy or perfect all the time, if ever. All people want is to hang out. That's really the best part of the meal.

THE LAST WORD

F. Scott Fitzgerald once said that "the test of a first-rate intelligence is the ability to hold two opposed ideas in the mind at the same time, and still retain the ability to function. One should, for example, be able to see that things are hopeless and yet be determined to make them otherwise." [109]

More and more, it feels like we set the dinner table not just with food but with opposing ideas—tradition versus science, individuality versus community, and success versus happiness are just a few of the sides it seems we must either choose or balance to function in today's world. But despite the mixed messages about what and how to eat, it's not about choosing sides or even about balance. It's about seeing all perspectives as part of a single story.

As an example, although the optics in the first microscope and telescope were nearly identical, because one pointed down and one pointed up, the stories they told were completely polar. Neither was right nor wrong. Without both perspectives, we wouldn't have our current understanding of the world or universe. Opposing ideas often create fragmented agendas, but they can also complement one another when seen as essential parts of a bigger picture. We can use science to change and evolve without giving up basic traditions that keep us grounded. We can trust our intellect and our intuition. And maybe if we keep our

heads up while also keeping our heads down, we can begin to see life and sport in a more meaningful way.

Biju and I set out to write *Feed Zone Table* because our intuition told us that something was missing in the way we were thinking about food, health, and performance. For us, the conversation felt one-sided, both professionally and personally. We realized that as much as the athletes we worked with often felt isolated and disconnected from one another, we felt the same. Having always used food to connect with others, we knew there was something about family-style dinners that wasn't exclusive to the traditional nuclear family, something that could help all of us. It's taken a lengthy intellectual discussion to come to the conclusion that regardless of where any of us are in our lives—whether young or old, single or married, training for the Olympics or simply struggling with our weight—we are all just human. Biju and I wanted to remind ourselves and others that food, health, and performance are part of a bigger picture that also includes our family,

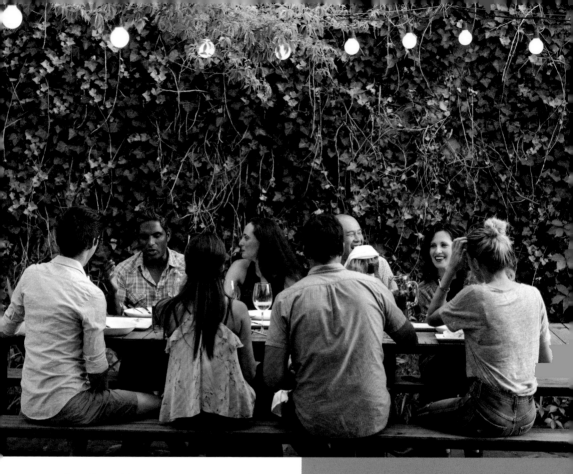

friends, and the greater community that surrounds us.

To that end, know that this cookbook only works if you use it. So pick a recipe, call a friend, set a date, go to the store, get in your kitchen, and share a meal. It doesn't have to be perfect. Despite what Yoda said, let's all just try. Let's try to make the table the center again—a place where one meal and one conversation have the potential to change ourselves and the world.

Bon appétit!

Allen

"Why is it that everything I eat when I'm with you is so delicious?" I laughed. "Could it be that you're satisfying hunger and lust at the same time?"

—Banana Yoshimoto, *Kitchen*

RECIPES

Cooking is a process—one that does not have to be a solitary chore, one that continuously evolves as we learn, and one that has its own reward and joy.

EAT & COOK

To become a good cook, you first have to be a good eater. This was easy for me, as I come from a large family of healthy eaters known to be obsessed with great-tasting food.

My mom's kitchen was always nice and hot on cold, snowy Colorado days as we crowded around her in anticipation of a steaming hot bowl of rice and spicy beef straight off the stove. To my mother's annoyance, all six of us kids would critique the dish and talk about how it was different from the last time, or how it would be so much better if we only toasted the onions a little longer, or charred the coconut, or added just a bit more broth. My mother would agree, and next time we would make it differently and the conversation would start all over again.

Being a good eater also requires that you cultivate a positive relationship with food. This can be tricky for athletes, who demand a lot from their bodies and rely on the foods they eat for both recovery and performance. It might explain why athletes generally fall into two camps: There are those who love to eat and those who agonize over the dos and don'ts of what to eat. In my experience, the pleasure of a home-cooked meal with friends is usually lost on those who take a more rigid, calorie-only approach to eating.

Throughout my career as a professional chef, I have cooked for countless athletes at different stages in their chase of a specific goal or outcome. Whatever their competition level, the successful athletes have a good relationship with food. Since we find ourselves needing to eat at least a couple of times each day, why not learn to love it? Not only will you see your performance improve while competing, you'll also build skills for creating a lifetime of delicious meals after training and competition.

Start by taking time to notice and appreciate how something tastes, the finer details of texture and color in the foods you love, and how you feel after you eat them. Some meals will make you feel alert, charged, and ready to take on anything, while other meals can be more calming, promoting rest and recovery. And unfortunately, there will inevitably be some foods that simply don't work— maybe they raise your body temperature, create stress or anxiety, or cause you to not feel well. It's impossible for every meal to be perfectly plated, full of flavor, and nourishing in all the right ways, but that's all part of the process. Although it might seem as if restaurant chefs effortlessly turn out perfect dishes every time, I can assure you that we have made something less than perfect a thousand times—each time we learn a simple thing that helps us to improve.

Remember that you are not building a precision rocket ship— you are just making dinner.

The recipes we have collected here are all meant to be flexible and not fussy. Even the most complicated-looking dish can be mastered with just a few tries. I've left room for you to adjust salt and acid levels up or down to your own taste with every dish. Remember that you are not building a precision rocket ship—you are just making dinner. Take some liberties: Use seasonal vegetables, change up the flavor, or save time by using a prepared sauce or dressing. I've tipped you off to some of these opportunities throughout the book.

Pick out the meals you enjoy most, the ones you are familiar with, and make those first. After you establish a number of go-to meals, try your hand at some of the more ambitious recipes—Baked Salmon in Pastry, Red Chicken with Baked Biriyani, and Allen's Ramen, to name a few. Don't wait for a special occasion or a holiday. Your time in the kitchen will be more fun if you keep expanding your repertoire of foods.

Above all else, I hope that the recipes in this book spark your imagination and get you into the kitchen so you can share more meals with your family and friends. Once this becomes part of your routine, the love takes over, regardless of what's being served for dinner. In my family, we were often eating a lot of steamed yucca and fried fish—humble staples in Indian culture. Even now the mere mention of *kappa* or *meen* makes me instantly hungry. It's the simple joy of gathering around the table to share stories over a home-cooked meal that will keep everyone coming back for more. Enjoy!

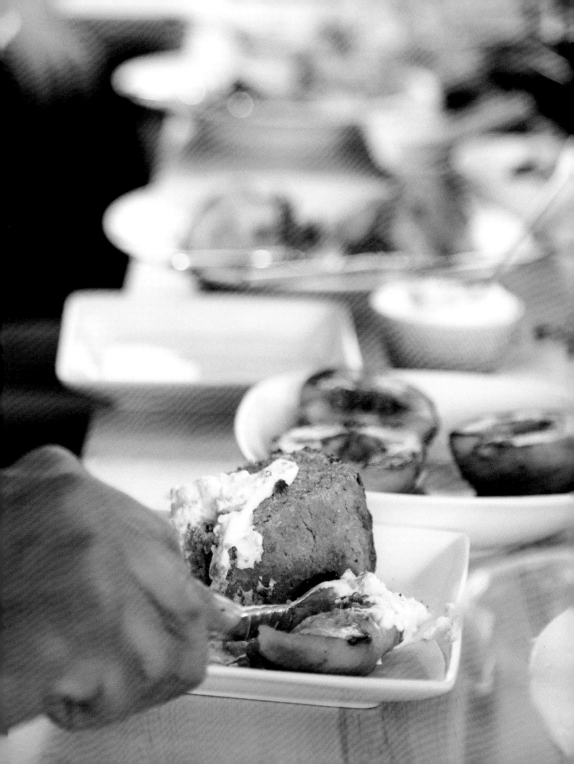

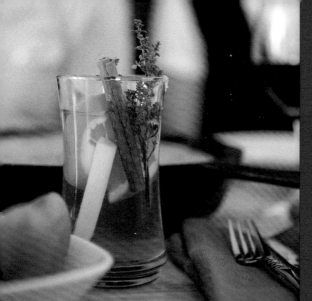

Allen remodeled his house around the dinner table. Previously, his 900-square-foot condo could barely accommodate four people for dinner. Having a place for everyone to sit improves both health and happiness.

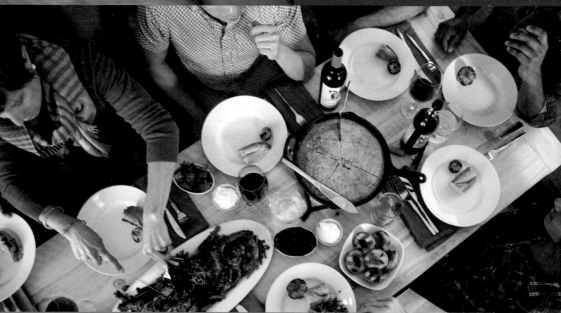

SET THE TABLE

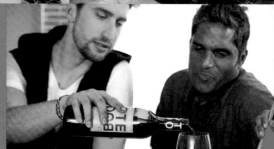

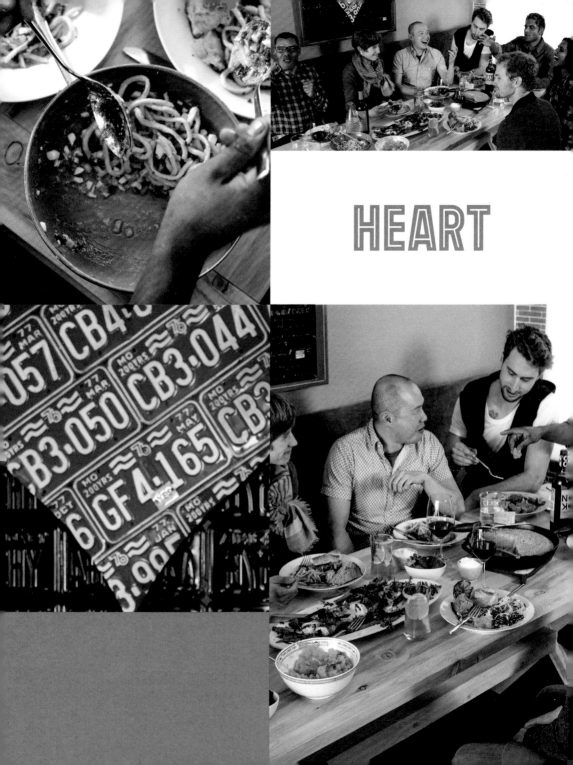

HEART

BE FESTIVE

*Whatever the season, it's fun to raise a glass with
friends and family. Give a classic beverage new flair with
a special garnish, some bubbles, or real fruit juice.*

DRINKS

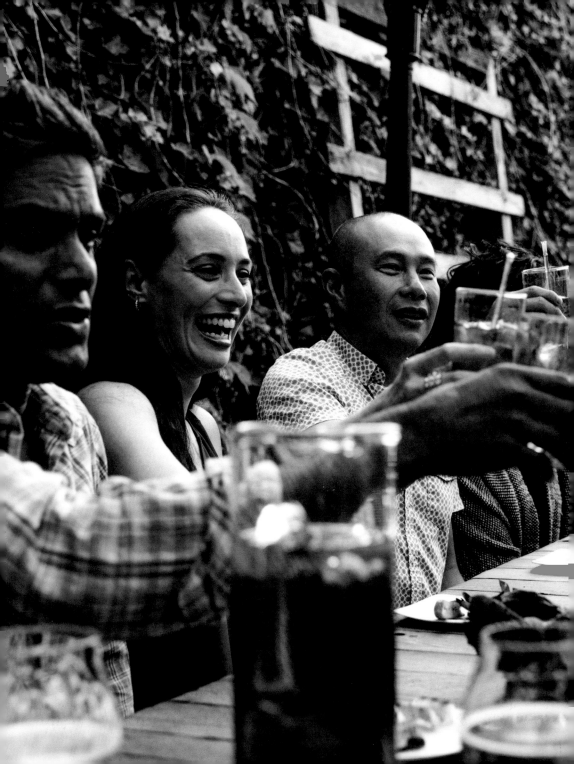

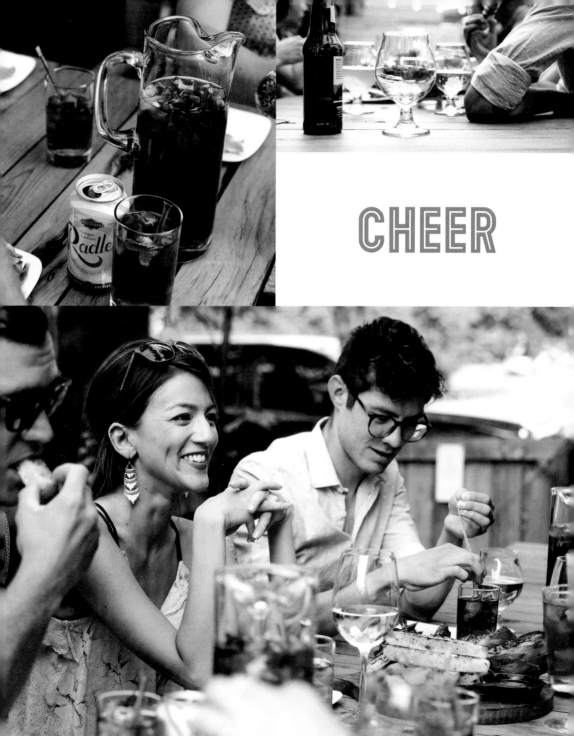

CHEER

LEMON HIBISCUS ICED TEA WITH HONEY

This is a beautiful and colorful tea with a refreshing touch of lemon. It's wonderful during the warmer months, for picnics and grilling outside. I like to use a blend of teas—the black tea gives it body and the hibiscus tea brings light floral flavors and nice color. Adjust the recipe to brew enough for a large crowd—simply use one tea bag of each variety for every two servings. • Most grocery stores sell a mix of edible flowers that you can find next to fresh herbs—pansies, nasturtiums, snapdragons, or rose petals. Check to see what is locally available to you. **Serves 6**

3 cups water
3 bags black tea
3 bags hibiscus tea
2 tablespoons honey or agave
　　syrup or 6 honey sticks
3 cups cold water
1 lemon, cut in half lengthwise
　　and sliced thin
handful of fresh mint
handful of edible flowers

Heat the water in a saucepan until it comes to a simmer.

Add the tea bags and let steep for 5 minutes. The tea will take on a deep ruby-red color when it is ready. Remove tea bags. If you are using honey or agave syrup, stir it in while the tea is still hot. Pour in the cold water and let the tea cool in the refrigerator while you are making dinner.

Just before serving, pour over ice and slivers of lemon and garnish with fresh mint and edible flowers. Cut the tops off the honey sticks, if using, and place in individual glasses cut-side up.

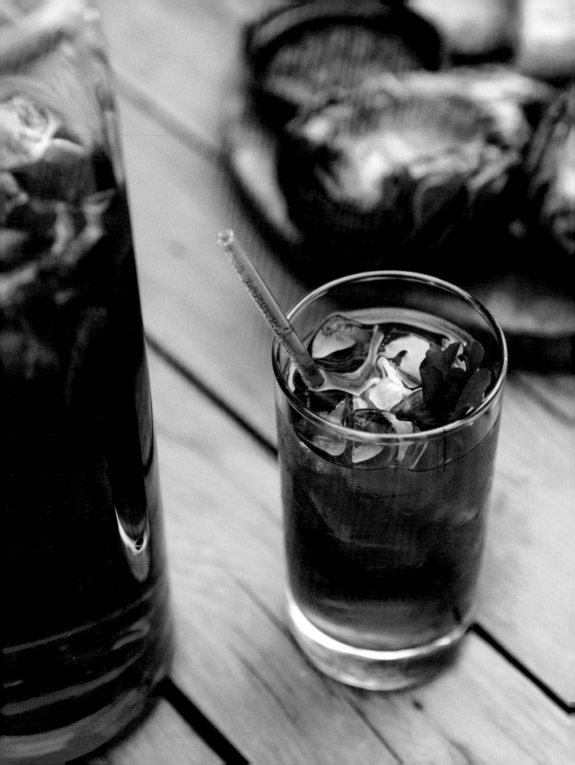

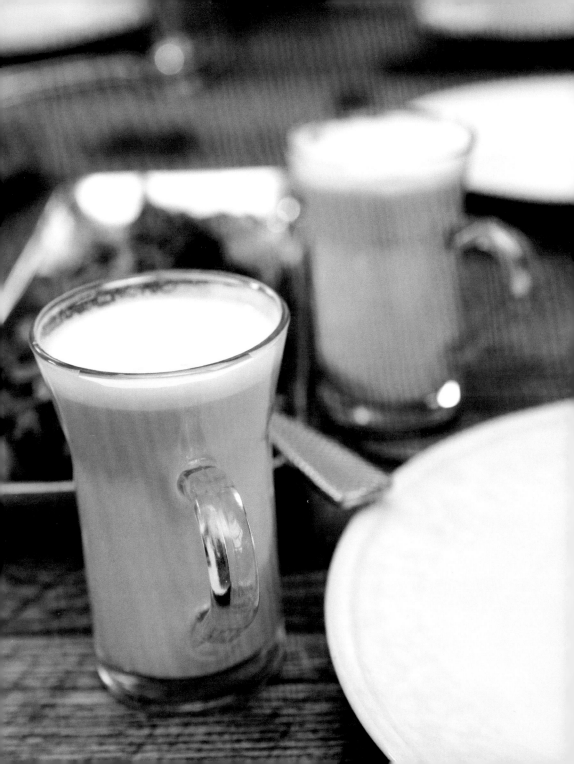

MUMBAI SPICED CHAI

This is my single most favorite beverage from my childhood home, India. The spices used and the strength of the tea vary from region to region, but the basics of a good chai are simple: a strong black tea (Assam, Ceylon, or pekoe), your favorite milk, and a touch of sweetness. From there you can add in any number of spices that make you happy. **Serves 6**

3 cups water
6 tea bags or 6 tablespoons
   loose-leaf black tea
3 cinnamon sticks
1 thumb fresh ginger, smashed
2 cloves cardamom
½ teaspoon whole black
   peppercorns
6 teaspoons brown sugar,
   honey, or agave
3 cups milk
sprinkle of cinnamon

In a tea kettle, bring the water to a boil. While the water is heating, place the tea and spices in a saucepan. Pour the boiling water over them.

Steep the tea until it is nice and strong, about 5–10 minutes. Squeeze out the tea bags (if using) and strain the liquid. Stir in sweetener of your choice and milk while the mixture is still warm.

For an iced chai, let cool and pour over ice.

For a hot chai, return the chai to the saucepan and bring to a low simmer. Be sure to stir the liquid to keep the milk from scorching.

Top with a sprinkle of cinnamon and drink it down.

TASTES GREAT BEFORE OR AFTER ENJOYING RED CHICKEN & BAKED BIRIYANI (P. 170).

SPICED APPLE CIDER

The problem with spiced apple cider is that all of the good stuff—cinnamon sticks, ginger, citrus—usually stays in the pot and I find myself holding a mug of plain old cider. Still good, but not nearly as great as having that goodness in my mug. I've gone overboard on the garnish for this festive drink—consider buying lots more cider because there's enough flavor in the mug for an evening of refills. **Serves 6**

6 cups apple cider
1 thumb fresh ginger, peeled
6 cinnamon sticks
1 orange, sliced into rounds
6 sprigs fresh thyme

RIM TOPPER
2 tablespoons coarse sugar
1 teaspoon cinnamon

In a heavy pot over medium-high heat, bring the apple cider to a low simmer.

TO MAKE THE RIM TOPPER: Mix together coarse sugar and cinnamon on a small plate. Use an orange slice to wet the lip of each glass. Twist each glass through the mixture until it is lightly coated.

TO MAKE THE GARNISH: Cut the ginger into long pieces about the same size as the cinnamon sticks and gently press (this makes it more flavorful). Place one piece of ginger and one cinnamon stick into each individual glass along with a slice of orange and a sprig of thyme.

Place any extra garnish in the pot of cider. Pour the hot apple cider into individual glasses just before serving.

Note: To enjoy this as a post-workout beverage, use Apples & Cinnamon Exercise Hydration Mix from Skratch Labs in place of cider.

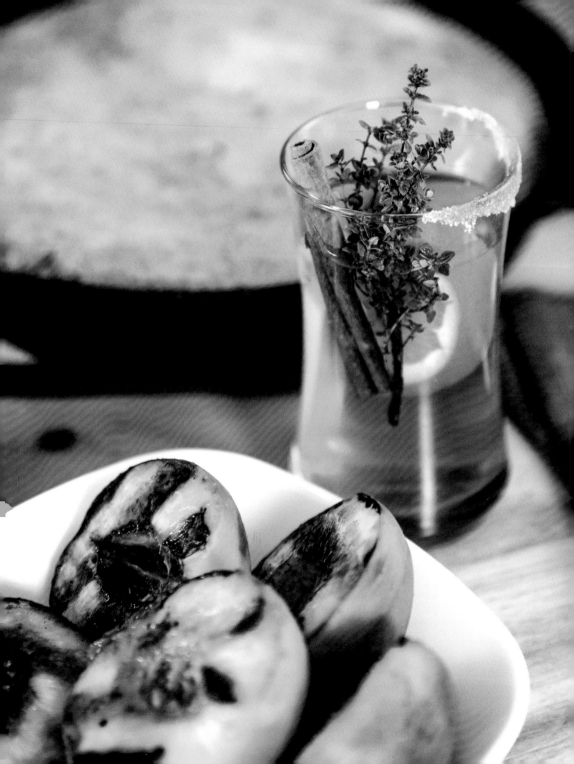

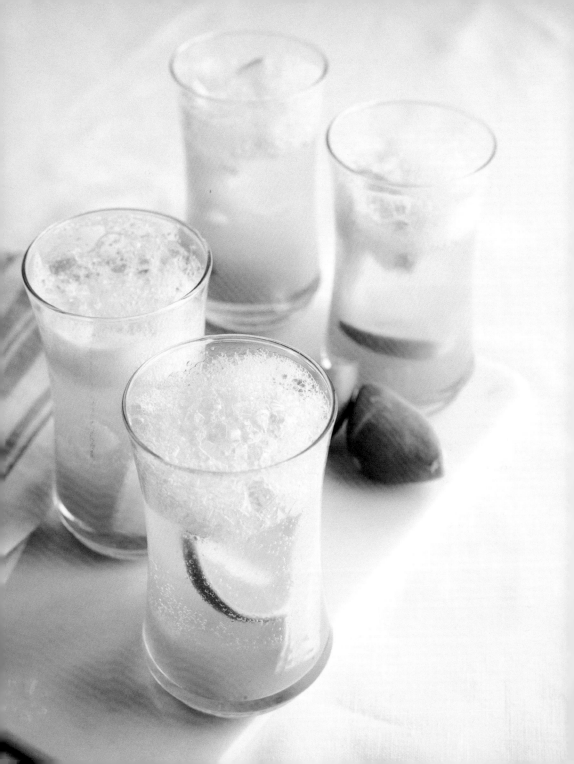

SALTY CUCUMBER LIME SODA

On a really hot day you often find yourself craving salt, and drinks like this one replenish the salt lost in sweat. It's a light soda reminiscent of drinks commonly served in more tropical parts of the world. In South India, where I grew up, you would also likely see green mango used. In fact, that was the inspiration for the Skratch Labs Hyper Hydration Mix with Mangos. Here I chose fresh cucumber, another delicious flavor that is both inexpensive and available year-round. **Serves 6**

2 cups cold water
1 medium cucumber,
    partially peeled lengthwise
    and cut in half
juice from 1 lime, plus
    additional to taste
quarter of a lime, peel on
    (reserve the rest for garnish)
2 tablespoons coarse sugar
    dissolved in 1 tablespoon hot
    water
1 teaspoon coarse salt
4 cups soda water

GARNISH
1 teaspoon coarse salt
1 teaspoon coarse sugar
remaining lime, sliced
remaining half cucumber,
    cut into long wedges

TO MAKE A SUGAR-SALT RIM: Mix together the salt and sugar. Run a lime slice along the rim of each glass, then twist it in the salt and sugar mixture until lightly coated.

TO MAKE THE SODA: In a blender, combine the water, half of the cucumber, lime juice, lime quarter, dissolved sugar, and salt. Pulse until the lime quarter is completely broken down.

Fill glasses with ice and a cucumber wedge. Pour the juice mixture through a mesh strainer to fill individual glasses half full. Top off with soda water and a slice of lime.

WATERMELON SODA WITH FRESH MINT

Watermelon is thought to speed recovery, making it the perfect finish to a hard summer-time ride. A good drink doesn't have to be complicated, and I think you'll find that this simple beverage has the power to please a lot of people quickly. It's a favorite of mine for its happy pink color, and the fact that it is naturally sweet. You'll also find it doubles as a great base for your favorite cocktails. **Serves 6**

4 cups of seedless watermelon, cut into chunks
6 cups soda water, divided
2–3 sprigs of fresh mint

Fill individual glasses halfway with ice.

Combine the watermelon with 1 cup of soda water in a blender and blend until all of the chunks break down. Pour the watermelon mixture through a mesh strainer and into individual glasses. Top off with remaining soda water and garnish with fresh mint.

Slivers of watermelon make a great garnish.

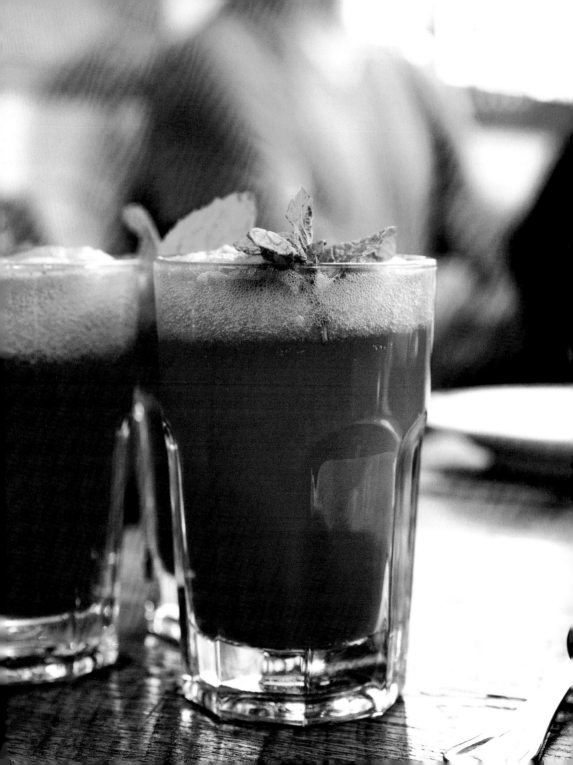

VIETNAMESE-STYLE COFFEE

Sometimes a caffeine kick is the perfect end to a meal. Vietnamese coffee typically calls for sweetened condensed milk, which is loaded with sugar. By using plain Greek yogurt, you can make a delicious, protein-rich beverage. The quintessential ingredient is chicory coffee, which is as strong as it is dark in color. Chicory is roasted, ground, and mixed with the coffee. It's the root of bitter lettuce varieties such as endive that ironically balance out bold coffee flavor with a floral sweetness. • Look for Café Du Monde or French-style chicory coffee at your local grocery store. **Serves 4**

3 cups water
¼ cup ground chicory coffee
   (New Orleans style)
2 cups milk
1 cup plain Greek yogurt
1 tablespoon honey or
   maple syrup
¼ teaspoon vanilla extract

Start by brewing the coffee. Use about half as much coffee as you normally would because it brews up strong. A conventional coffeemaker works just fine, but a French press comes close to replicating authentic Vietnamese coffee, which typically is made using individual filters that sit on top of individual cups. If you are using a coffee press, boil the water, then pour over the grounds and let brew for about 4 minutes. Let cool to room temperature.

In a small mixing bowl, gently whisk the milk, Greek yogurt, honey or maple syrup, and vanilla until smooth, then split between 4 cups. Once the coffee has cooled, gently pour it over the yogurt and milk mixture. The drink will settle into two distinct layers. Serve with a spoon.

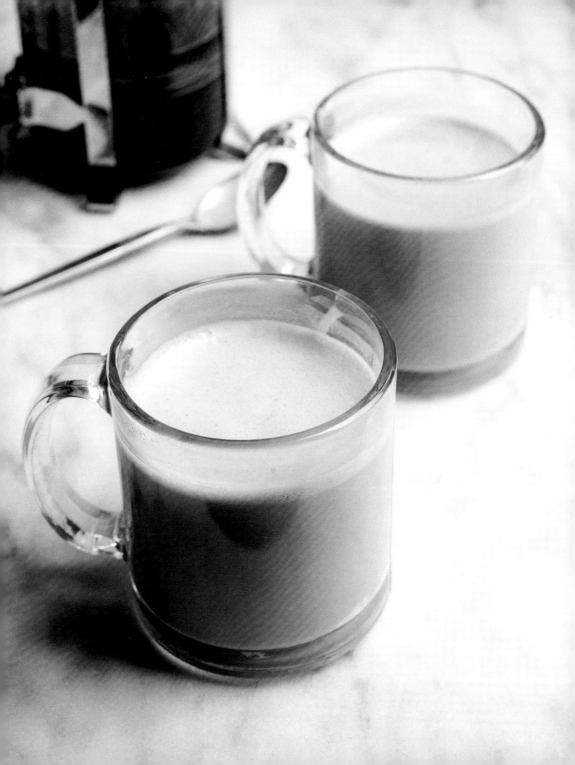

SPARKLING GINGER SODA

This is a fizzy drink with a bright burst of juiced ginger—it's the perfect match for more hearty dishes. You definitely need a juicer to do the job of separating the ginger pulp from the juice. Because fresh ginger is so intense and peppery, start with just a little bit. You might just find yourself coming back for more. **Serves 6**

1 cup water
½ cup coarse sugar
4 big thumbs fresh ginger
6 cups club soda or
    sparkling water
1 orange or lemon,
    cut in half and sliced thin

In a small pot over medium-high heat, bring the water and sugar to a low simmer until the sugar is fully dissolved to make simple syrup. (You can also substitute 1 cup agave nectar or maple syrup for the simple syrup.)

Peel the ginger root and put it in a juicer to extract the liquid.

Mix together equal parts ginger juice and simple syrup. (If you have leftover simple syrup, save it for another round of drinks.)

Fill individual glasses three-quarters full with ice cubes, club soda or sparkling water, and orange or lemon slices, then top off with the ginger simple syrup to taste.

SERVE WITH ASIAN-INSPIRED DISHES LIKE KIMCHEE SPICED SALAD (P. 127) AND ALLEN'S RAMEN (P. 221).

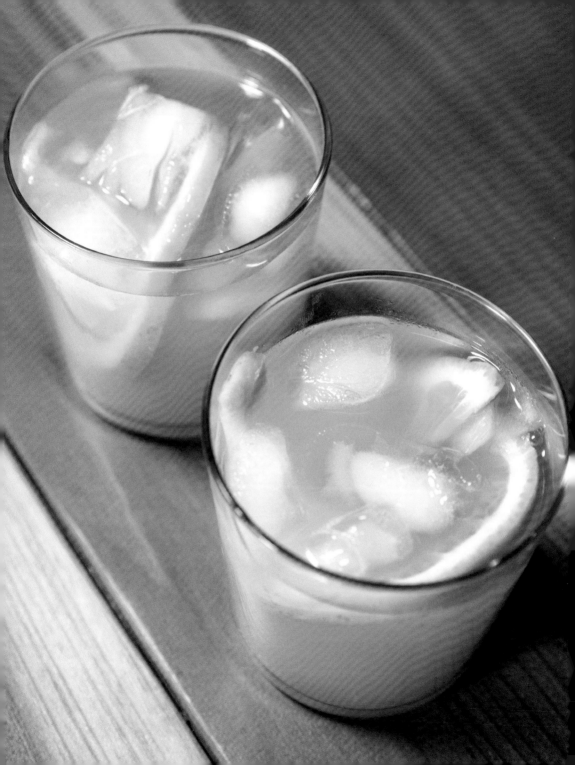

SWISS MOUNTAIN HERB TEA

Herbal liquors are known for helping to settle the stomach following a big meal. This warm beverage—with its fresh, bright flavors—will do just that, so serve it after dinner. Start with a black tea (this recipe uses a half-strength tea to let the herbal flavor come through) and add sprigs of rosemary and thyme to individual glasses to serve up that herbal menthol goodness we all love. **Serves 6**

6 cups water
3 tea bags or 3 heaping
   tablespoons loose-leaf
   black tea
2–3 fresh or dried rose hips
   (optional)
2 sprigs rosemary
2 sprigs thyme
2 teaspoons dried
   lavender buds
1 orange, sliced
1 lemon, sliced
honey to taste

Bring water to a boil. Remove from heat and add the black tea, rose hips (if you have them), 1–2 sprigs of rosemary and thyme, and dried lavender buds. Steep for at least 5 minutes—longer for a stronger flavor.

Remove the tea bags and pour into individual mugs and garnish with slices of citrus, more fresh herbs, and a drizzle of honey to taste.

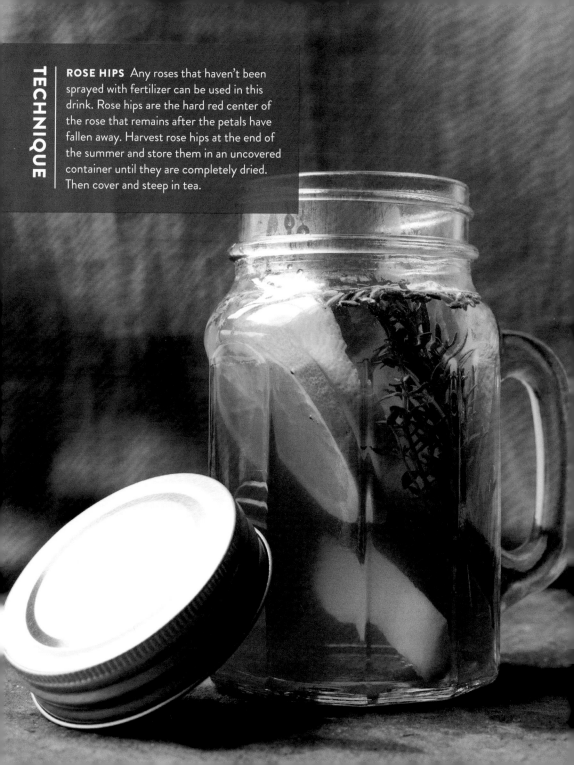

TECHNIQUE

ROSE HIPS Any roses that haven't been sprayed with fertilizer can be used in this drink. Rose hips are the hard red center of the rose that remains after the petals have fallen away. Harvest rose hips at the end of the summer and store them in an uncovered container until they are completely dried. Then cover and steep in tea.

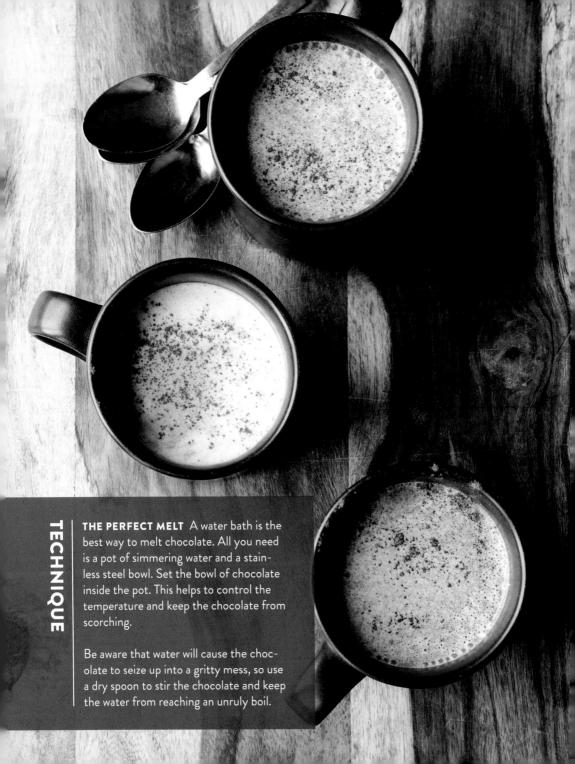

TECHNIQUE

THE PERFECT MELT A water bath is the best way to melt chocolate. All you need is a pot of simmering water and a stainless steel bowl. Set the bowl of chocolate inside the pot. This helps to control the temperature and keep the chocolate from scorching.

Be aware that water will cause the chocolate to seize up into a gritty mess, so use a dry spoon to stir the chocolate and keep the water from reaching an unruly boil.

HOMEMADE
HOT CHOCOLATE

The notion of chocolate milk as a recovery drink for athletes has enjoyed a fair amount of press in recent years. Some might argue about how effective it is, but I think we can all agree that hot chocolate can be a satisfying dessert for grown-ups. Made from scratch with bittersweet chocolate chips, it has less sugar and fewer calories than the typical chocolate desserts. I like mine with a splash of bourbon (for recovery). **Serves 4**

1 cup bittersweet chocolate
   chips
3 cups almond, soy,
   or dairy milk
1 teaspoon brown sugar,
   plus additional to taste
sprinkle of cinnamon

Fill a pot or skillet with 1 inch of water. Pour the chocolate chips into a heatproof bowl and set the bowl inside the pot. Bring the water to a simmer over medium-high heat.

As the chocolate begins to melt, stir occasionally until you have a smooth consistency. Remove from heat and empty the water from the pot.

Gently warm the milk in a pot over medium heat, stirring to keep it from scorching. Stir in the melted chocolate until it is fully incorporated. Stir in the brown sugar, adding more to taste if desired. The milk will froth up a bit as it reaches a simmer. Remove from heat and pour into individual mugs. Finish them off with a sprinkle of cinnamon.

TAKE A BITE

*Think of starters as part of the meal, not a meal before
the meal. Pick something that's easy to share, and
win over your friends and family from their very first bite.*

STARTERS

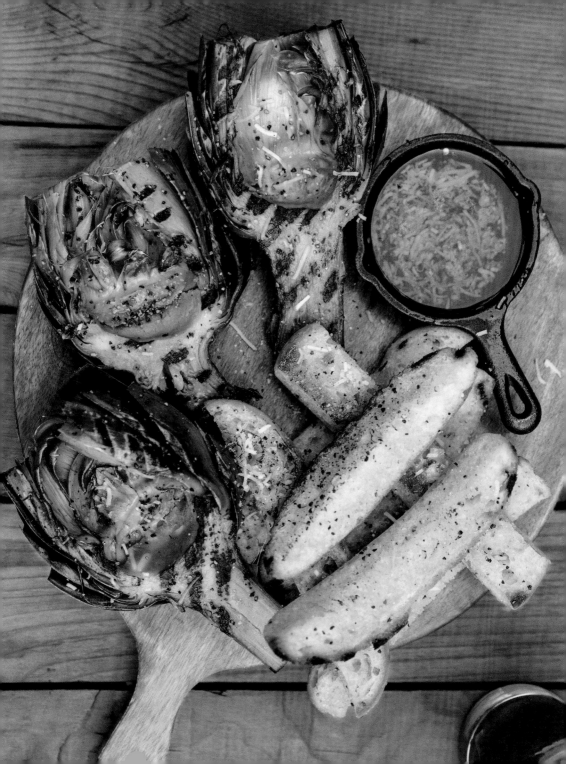

GRILLED BREAD & ARTICHOKES WITH DIPPING OIL

This appetizer serves the appetites of your more adventurous friends and family, as well as those who like to play it safe. Artichokes can be a little intimidating, but they are really simple to work with once you get your head around the basics. After steaming the artichokes, I like to finish them on the grill or sear at high heat to add some color and texture. **Serves 8**

4 artichokes
half a lemon, cut into wedges
1 baguette or any hearty bread
   (ciabatta works well)
2 tablespoons olive oil
coarse salt and pepper to taste
1 tablespoon freshly grated
   Parmesan

BALSAMIC DIPPING OIL
½ cup extra-virgin olive oil
2 tablespoons balsamic vinegar
juice from half a lemon,
   plus additional to taste

TO MAKE THE ARTICHOKES: Remove the tough leaves near the stem of the artichoke. Use kitchen shears to cut off the tip of each leaf (about ½ inch), removing the tiny needle. Trim the base of each stem and any dark spots with a sharp knife.

Fill a large stockpot three-quarters full of salted water. Bring to a boil over high heat and add artichokes along with the lemon wedges. Reduce heat to low, cover, and let simmer for about 30 minutes, or until the bottom leaves pull off easily and the artichokes feel tender to the touch. Drain the artichokes and set them aside to cool slightly.

TO MAKE THE BREAD STICKS: Cut the bread into long "sticks" and lightly brush with olive oil. Place on the grill or under the broiler and turn after 2 minutes. Toast for 1–2 minutes more, or until golden brown. Sprinkle with a bit of coarse salt while the bread is still warm and set aside until the artichokes are ready to serve.

TO MAKE THE DIPPING OIL: Mix together olive oil, vinegar, and lemon juice. Taste and adjust with additional lemon juice, if desired. Set aside.

(recipe continues)

TO FINISH THE ARTICHOKES: Cut each one in half and scoop out the fibrous center, otherwise known as the choke. The rest of the stem and the base of each leaf are edible and delicious. Brush each artichoke half with olive oil and grill cut-side down just long enough to get nice char marks.

(Alternatively, you can finish the artichokes on the stovetop in a large skillet over high heat.)

Arrange the artichokes and bread sticks on a large platter, and finish with coarsely ground pepper, a sprinkle of Parmesan, and a squeeze of lemon juice. Serve with the dipping oil.

PERFECT WITH GRILLED CHICKEN WITH HOMEMADE BARBECUE SAUCE (P. 160).

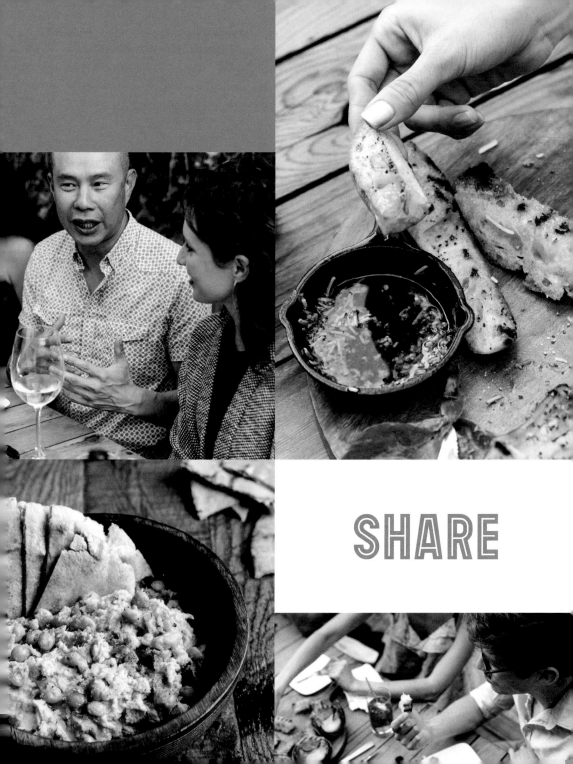

SHARE

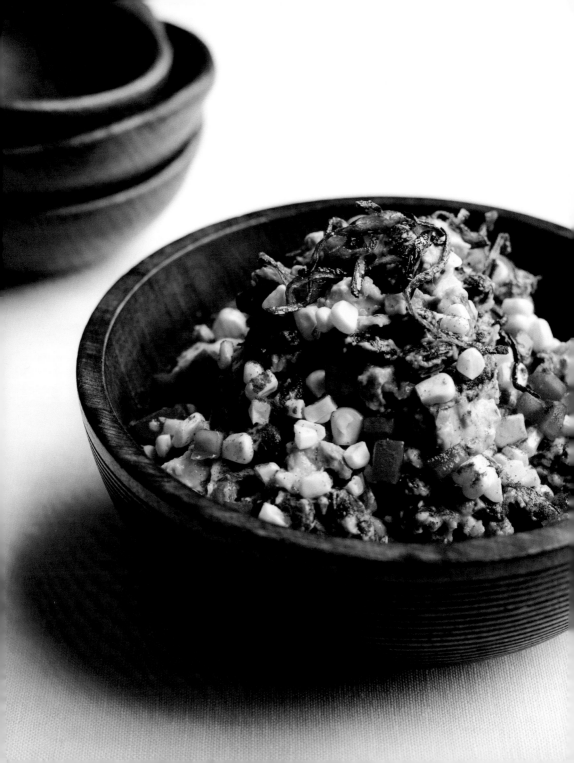

GUACAMOLE
WITH BEANS

Kept chunky and rustic with red or black beans and chopped herbs, guacamole can be a bright salad packed with good fats and protein. High-quality beans are an economical way to feed more people. This is a crowd-pleaser that you can make last-minute and serve at room temperature. **Serves 8**

3 ripe avocados, diced large
¼ cup finely diced red onion
¼ cup chopped fresh
    cilantro leaves
1 tablespoon diced jalapeño
juice from half a lime, plus
    additional to taste
1 cup canned or cooked red
    kidney beans or black beans
1 teaspoon chili powder
salt and pepper to taste

ON TOP
¼ cup thinly sliced onion,
    sautéed until crisp
1 ear of fresh sweet corn
1 small tomato, diced
1 tablespoon extra-virgin
    olive oil to drizzle
crumbled fresh milk cheese:
    farmer cheese, queso
    fresco, or feta (optional)

In a medium-sized mixing bowl, combine the avocados, red onion, cilantro, jalapeño, and half the lime juice.

If you are using canned beans, drain and rinse them before folding into the guacamole. Mix in the chili powder, salt, and pepper, being careful not to crush the beans.

Taste and add more lime juice and salt and pepper, if needed. Sprinkle with any combination of toppers and serve immediately.

ITALIAN RICE BALLS WITH RED PEPPER OIL & LEMON PESTO

Also known as arancini, these rice balls are the perfect fare for a large gathering. You can also serve them as a carbohydrate boost to a fresh green salad. You'll want to use fresh-cooked, warm rice, which helps the rice balls stick together. **Serves 8**

2 cups uncooked short-grain rice (short-grain brown rice works well)
1 cup ricotta
1 tablespoon freshly grated Parmesan
2 eggs, lightly beaten
¼ cup chopped fresh Italian herbs (basil, tarragon, thyme, parsley)
zest from half a lemon
1 teaspoon salt
1 egg plus 1 tablespoon water, lightly beaten
1 cup gluten-free panko or bread crumbs
½ cup olive oil

ON TOP
freshly grated Parmesan

RED PEPPER OIL
1 red bell pepper
2 tablespoons extra-virgin olive oil
coarse salt to taste

Prepare the rice in a rice cooker or on the stovetop, following the instructions on the package.

TO MAKE THE RED PEPPER OIL: While the rice is cooking, blanch the bell pepper in salted boiling water for no more than 1 minute. The skin will be wrinkled. Run the pepper under cold water, then peel off the skin and remove the stem and seeds. Place the pepper in a blender with the olive oil and purée. Season to taste with coarse salt and set aside.

TO MAKE THE RICE BALLS: Heat the oven to 250 degrees. Once the cooked rice is cool enough to handle, transfer it into a large bowl and add the ricotta, Parmesan, eggs, herbs, lemon zest, and salt. Mix together with a wooden spoon. It will be sticky. Shape into large, firm balls, about 2 inches in diameter (the size of a golf ball). Makes about 32 rice balls. Brush egg and water mixture onto each rice ball, then roll in the bread crumbs.

In large sauté pan or skillet over medium-high heat, heat the olive oil, then add the rice balls in batches. Don't crowd the pan. Turn frequently until golden brown on all sides. Each batch will take about 8–10 minutes to cook. Transfer to a baking sheet and keep warm in the oven while you finish making the remaining rice balls. Add more olive oil if needed.

Pile the rice balls on a serving platter and top with freshly grated Parmesan. Serve with red pepper oil, pesto (see p. 80 for Lemon Pesto), or your favorite marinara.

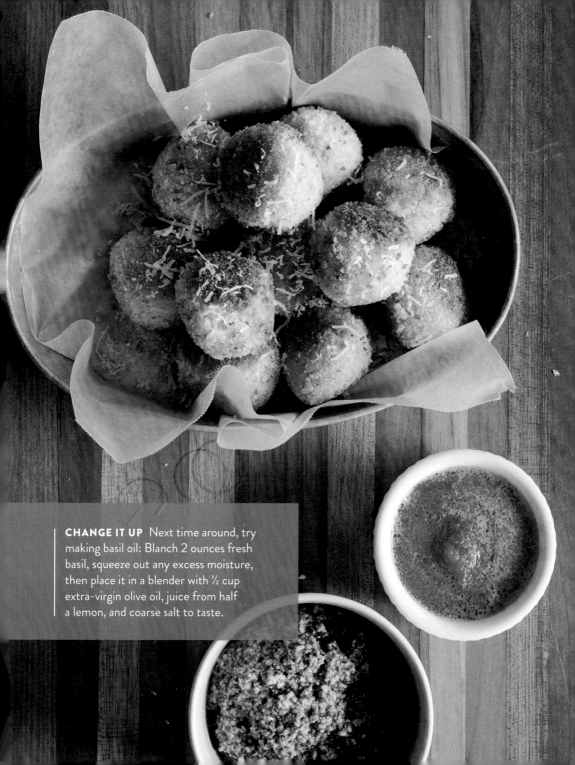

CHANGE IT UP Next time around, try making basil oil: Blanch 2 ounces fresh basil, squeeze out any excess moisture, then place it in a blender with ½ cup extra-virgin olive oil, juice from half a lemon, and coarse salt to taste.

Lemon Pesto

I don't want you to miss out on the extra flavor this pesto delivers—make it in advance so you don't run out of time. Add pesto to your pasta salads or just spread on toast and top with fresh tomatoes. **Makes 1 cup**

2 cups fresh basil, loosely
   packed
2 garlic cloves, minced
½ cup pine nuts or walnuts
1 tablespoon freshly grated
   Parmesan
½ cup extra-virgin olive oil,
   plus additional to taste
juice from 1 lemon,
   plus additional to taste
salt to taste

Combine basil, garlic, nuts, Parmesan, and olive oil in a food processor and pulse until smooth. Season to taste: If it's too acidic, add more olive oil. Add more lemon juice to brighten the flavor, and salt as needed.

Refrigerate unused pesto in a covered container for up to 1 week.

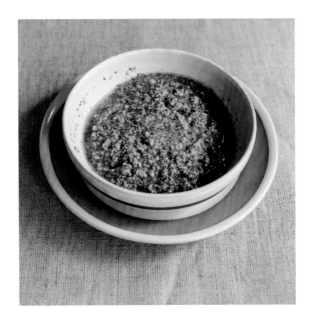

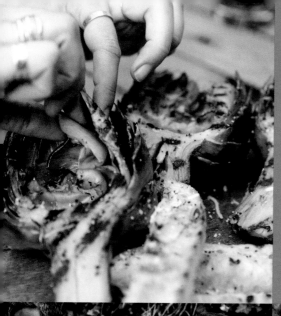

One of the great things about starters is that your guests will often be willing to taste food that they typically avoid. Make food that inspires your guests to bend the rules a little.

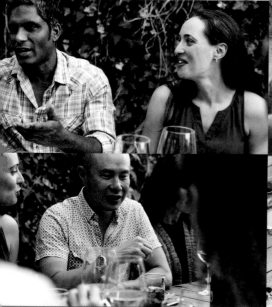

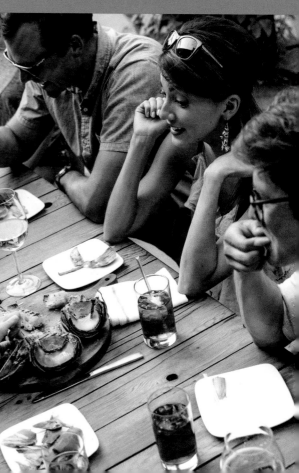

TAKE A BITE

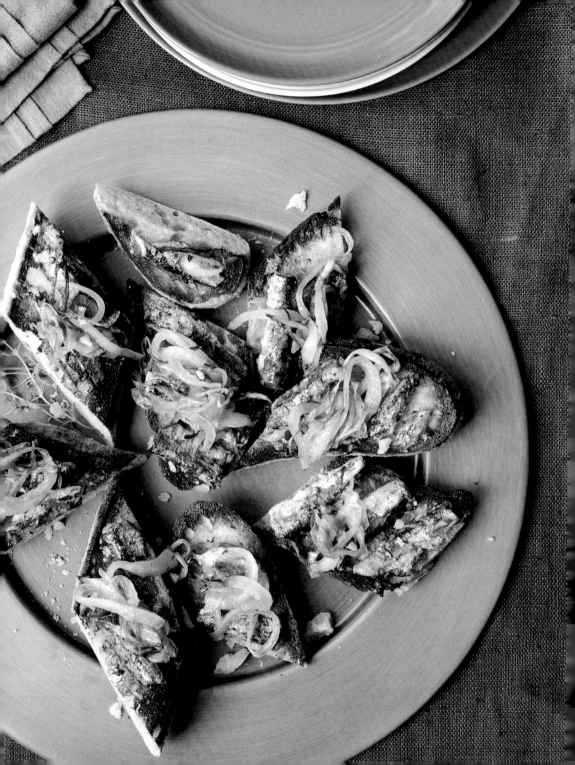

WHITE ANCHOVY TOAST

This is a great appetizer or snack to surprise your friends with your kitchen skills. Anchovies are nutrient-dense and flavorful—a good break from the ordinary. • Look for white anchovies at the fish counter. They are particularly mild and delicate . . . not the overly salted version that most people think of. If you can't find white anchovies, choose a tin of good-quality flat-packed anchovies in olive oil. **Serves 8**

1 tablespoon olive oil
½ cup thinly sliced onion
4 garlic cloves, sliced thin
1 loaf rustic bread, split
   lengthwise
4 ounces white anchovies

ON TOP
freshly grated Parmesan
coarsely ground black pepper
   to taste
extra-virgin olive oil to drizzle

Begin by caramelizing the onions: Heat the olive oil in a sauté pan over medium-high heat and add the onions and garlic. Cook until the onions are soft and slightly golden. Set aside.

The bread can be toasted on a hot grill or under the broiler. Turn the broiler on high and position the rack in the middle of the oven. Place the bread cut-side up on a baking sheet and broil it just long enough for the edges to char a little (no more than a couple of minutes—stand by so it doesn't burn).

Remove the bread from the oven and layer on the anchovies. Top with onions and garlic. Sprinkle with Parmesan and black pepper and finish with a little bit of olive oil.

TOASTED CHICKPEAS WITH GHOST PEPPER SALT

This snack has become popular with some of our athletes over the past few years. Ghost Pepper Salt packs a surprising amount of heat—the kind that sneaks up on you, starting from your shoulders and moving right up your neck. While it can be crazy hot, in the right balance Ghost Pepper Salt has an intensely warm, ethereal effect. It's a finishing spice that goes great with eggs and your favorite rice dishes. **Serves 4**

1 15-ounce can chickpeas or 2 cups cooked chickpeas
1 tablespoon coconut oil, melted
1 teaspoon Ghost Pepper Salt Mix

GHOST PEPPER SALT MIX
¼ cup coarse salt
1 tablespoon coarse sugar
1 teaspoon coriander
½ teaspoon cinnamon
1 teaspoon chili powder
¼ teaspoon ground ghost pepper (you can add as much as you'd like, but start here)

Heat the oven to 375 degrees.

If you are using canned chickpeas, drain and rinse them under cool water.

Spread chickpeas out on a baking sheet to let dry thoroughly while you make the spice mix.

Use a spoon to gently mix the Ghost Pepper Salt Mix ingredients together without creating dust.

Once the chickpeas are dry, toss them in the coconut oil in a medium-sized bowl. Transfer back to the baking sheet and place in the oven for approximately 5 minutes.

Gently shake the pan to loosen the chickpeas and turn them to their uncooked sides, then continue baking for another 10 minutes. Once they are toasty and brown, remove from the oven and generously sprinkle on the Ghost Pepper Salt while the chickpeas are still warm, then set aside and wait for your friends to show up!

Store the unused Ghost Pepper Salt Mix in an airtight container for future use.

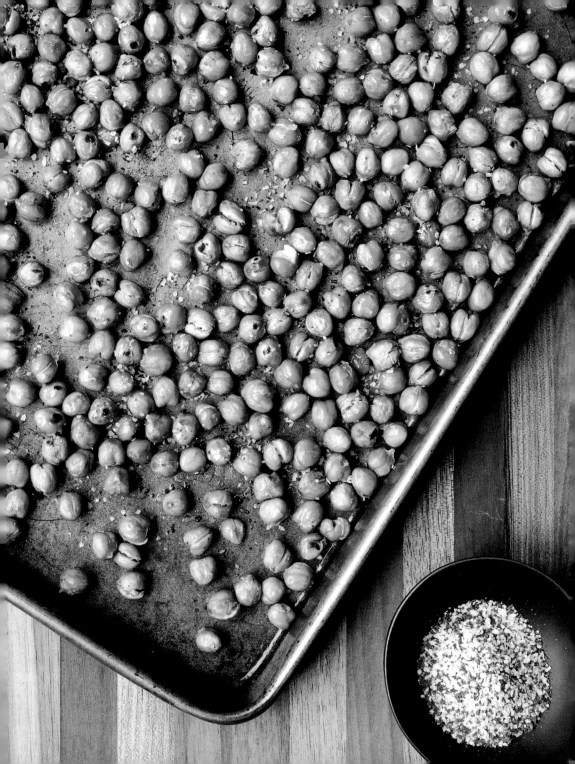

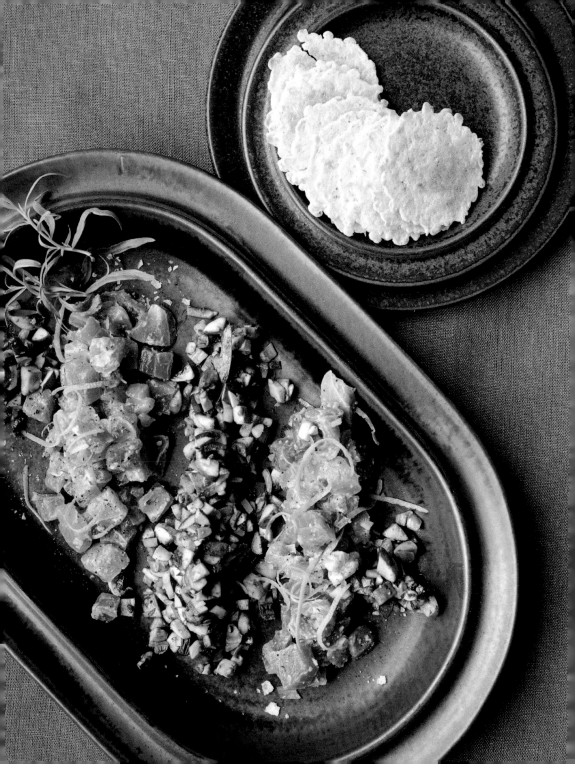

TUNA MUSHROOM SALAD WITH LEMON TARRAGON DRESSING

Good-quality tuna can be expensive, but served as an appetizer it is a wonderful dish to share with friends and family. **Serves 8**

1 pound fresh ahi tuna steak
4 ounces brown button
  mushrooms, diced

LEMON TARRAGON DRESSING
juice from 2 lemons
2 tablespoons extra-virgin
  olive oil
1 tablespoon white wine
  vinegar or rice vinegar
1 teaspoon minced
  fresh ginger
1 teaspoon honey
1 tablespoon chopped fresh
  tarragon, plus extra for
  garnish
zest from half a lemon
salt and pepper to taste

TO MAKE THE SALAD: Using a really sharp knife, trim off any white or dark parts of the fish to start with a ruby-red fresh tuna steak. Cut against the grain to make ½-inch-thick slices, then dice each slice.

Wash and then dice the mushrooms to approximately the same size as the tuna. Set aside while you make the dressing, keeping the two ingredients separate.

TO MAKE THE DRESSING: In a blender, combine the lemon juice, olive oil, vinegar, ginger, honey, and tarragon and pulse until smooth.

Just before serving, dress the mushrooms and tuna separately, using half of the dressing for the mushrooms and the other half for the tuna. Garnish with lemon zest and additional tarragon and season to taste with salt and pepper.

BITTER CHARD ON GRILLED BREAD

Simply grill or toast some bread and add these delicious toppings to enjoy this tasty appetizer. You can split a baguette lengthwise, pile everything on, and cut before serving. The acidity of the lemon juice and olive oil softens the chard without cooking it, making this the perfect appetizer for entertaining. It will be messy . . . and delicious. **Serves 6**

6 thick slices of rustic bread or one long half of a baguette
3 tablespoons olive oil, divided
1 cup walnuts
½ cup orange marmalade
¼ cup blue cheese crumbles
1 bunch (8 ounces) rainbow chard, stems removed and coarsely chopped
juice from half a lemon
salt and pepper to taste

Heat the grill to medium. Brush the bread with 1 tablespoon olive oil and simply warm the bread on the grill for about 5 minutes. (You can also toast the bread on the stovetop in a hot pan or under the broiler for just a few minutes. Watch closely to avoid burning the bread.)

While the bread is being prepared, toast the walnuts in a dry pan over medium-high heat, stirring frequently until color darkens and nuts become fragrant.

Smear the marmalade on the grilled bread and top with blue cheese crumbles.

In a large bowl, toss the chard and walnuts with the lemon juice, the remaining 2 tablespoons of olive oil, salt, and pepper until well coated. Pile the chard on top of the bread and serve.

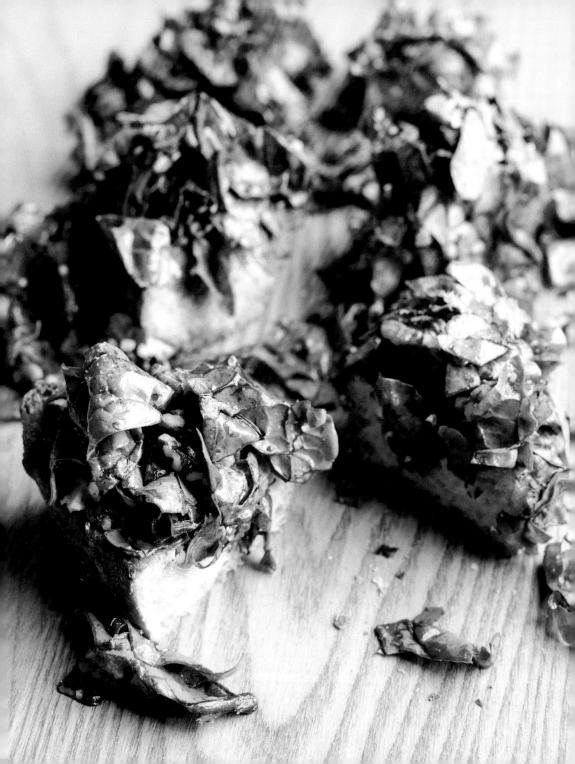

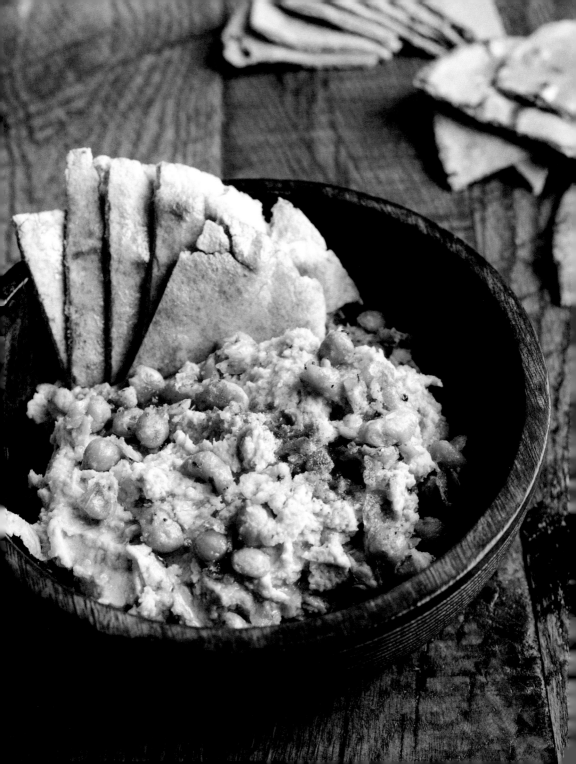

CLASSIC HUMMUS

Hummus you buy at the store is so smooth that you might forget that it is full of chickpeas. It's difficult to replicate that at home, so I like to play to my strengths and make it even more rustic. By toasting up some of the chickpeas, you can enhance both the flavor and the texture in hummus. After all, chickpeas are the hero of this modest dish. **Serves 4**

1 15-ounce can chickpeas or 2 cups cooked chickpeas, divided
1 tablespoon tahini (sesame paste)
3 tablespoons extra-virgin olive oil, divided
juice from 1 lemon, divided
½ teaspoon coarse salt, plus additional to taste
pepper and red pepper flakes to taste
½ teaspoon cayenne pepper (for a milder flavor, use sweet paprika)

If using canned chickpeas, drain and rinse them. Set aside ¼ cup for the topping. Combine the chickpeas with the tahini and 2 tablespoons olive oil in a small food processor and pulse until you have a smooth consistency. Incorporate half the lemon juice and the salt and adjust flavor as needed—add additional lemon juice for more acidity or olive oil if the flavor is too sharp. Transfer the hummus to a serving bowl.

In a dry sauté pan toast the remaining ¼ cup chickpeas over medium-high heat until golden brown. Add a drizzle of olive oil into the pan to crisp up the chickpeas. Then season with coarse salt, pepper, and red pepper flakes to taste and give it a gentle mash with a wooden spoon.

Top off the hummus with the toasted chickpeas, then sprinkle with the cayenne pepper or paprika, adding more to taste. Store in the refrigerator until ready to serve.

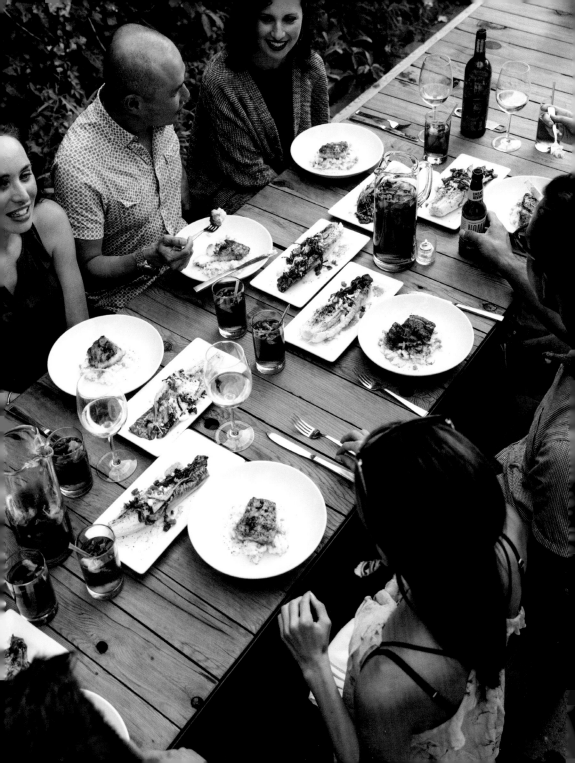

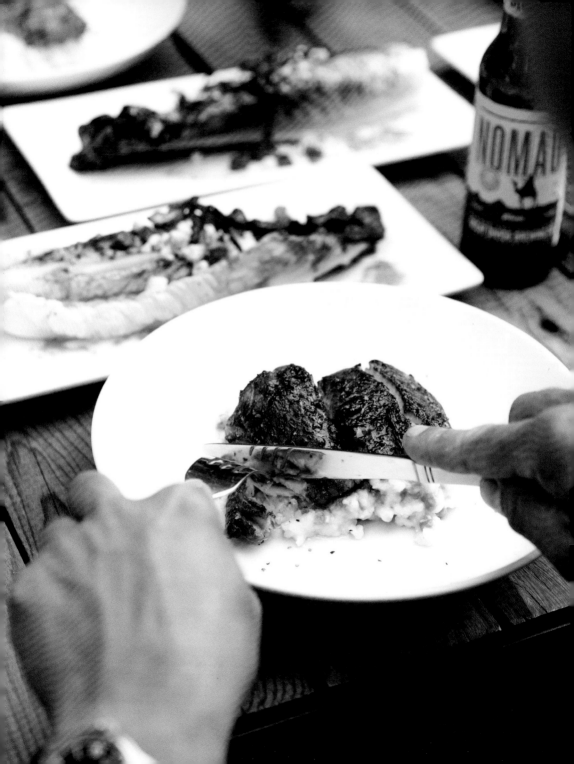

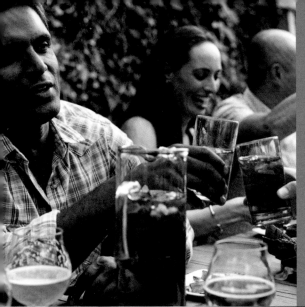

Keep a list of all the people you enjoy being around, and the next time you find yourself about to microwave a hot dog, invite a few of your friends over for dinner.

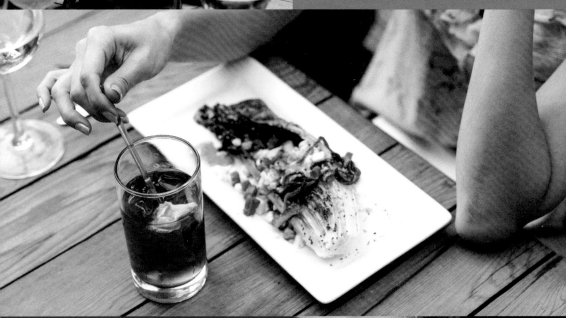

DON'T EAT ALONE

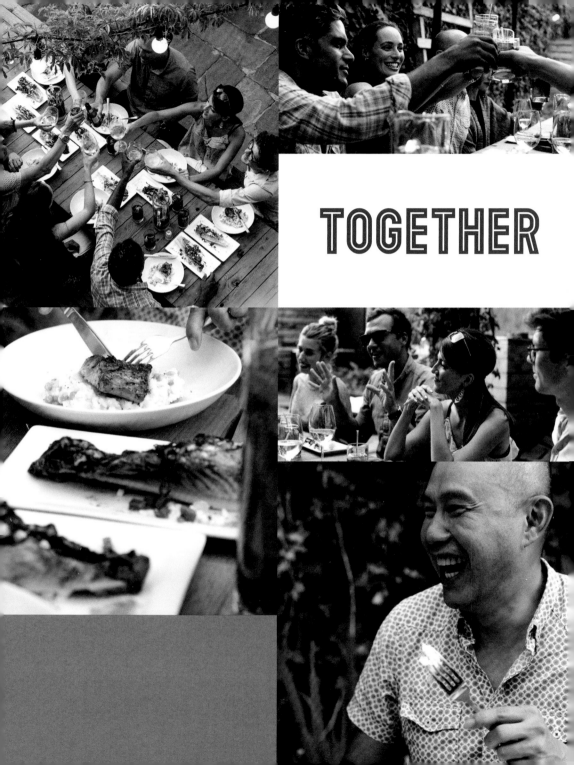

TOGETHER

THE STAPLES

*These recipes can be coupled up or paired with
a protein to make a great dinner. While the protein
is often the star of the table, what sits on the
side can be the most satisfying part of the meal.*

SIDES
SALADS
SOUPS

TECHNIQUE

BEEF BONE STOCK

You can use pretty much any vegetables you have on hand to make fresh stock. Just leave the skins and stalks on and put it all in a roasting pan. Pick up soup bones from an Asian market or your local grocer. If you don't have the time to wait around, put it all in the slow cooker—the flavor will still beat out store-bought stock. **Makes approximately 6 quarts**

3–4 pounds beef bones
3 large carrots
1 large onion
3 stalks celery
½ bulb garlic
½ bunch parsley, including stems
1 6-ounce can tomato paste
2 bay leaves
1 tablespoon peppercorns
3 sprigs fresh thyme
salt to taste
2 teaspoons dry herbs such as
    rosemary, tarragon, thyme
    (optional)
1 cup red wine

Heat the oven to 400 degrees.

Place the beef bones in a metal roasting pan. Chop the vegetables into large chunks without peeling them or removing any of the outer skin. Add the remaining ingredients, except the dry herbs and red wine. Toss everything together until the tomato paste lightly coats all of the vegetables. Put the pan on the top rack of the oven and roast for 1 hour, or until the bones and vegetables begin to blacken.

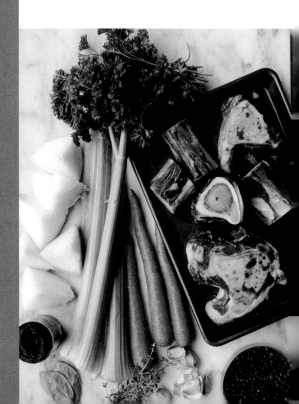

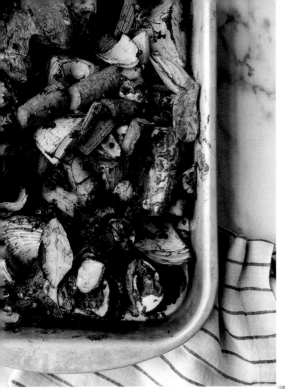

3

Strain the stock and store to use in your favorite soups and sauces. Homemade stock will keep for up to 1 week in the refrigerator. You can also freeze it in 1-quart bags.

2

Transfer all of the roasted bones and vegetables into an 8-quart stockpot or a slow cooker. Add dry herbs, if using. While the roasting pan is still hot, add red wine and use a spatula to deglaze the pan, scraping off all of the burnt and stuck pieces.

Put all of these flavorful bits into the stockpot and fill with water, up to 1 inch below the top of the pot. Bring the stock to a low rolling boil and simmer for about 5 hours. If you are using a slow cooker, set heat to low and cook overnight.

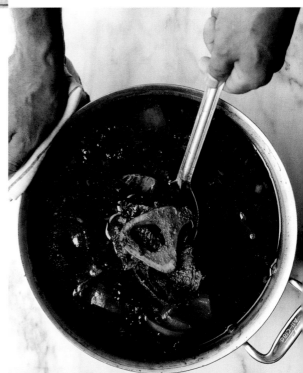

VEGETABLE STOCK

To make a good vegetable stock, start by saving up your scraps—carrot tops, onion trimmings, leafy parts of celery and root vegetables. You'll want to have about 4 cups in total. If you come up a little short, make up the difference with a mix of carrots, onion, and celery. **Makes approximately 4 quarts**

4 cups vegetable trimmings
  (or 3 large carrots, 1 large onion,
  and 3 stalks celery)
½ bulb garlic, unpeeled and
  slightly smashed
1 bunch parsley, including stems
3–4 stems fresh herbs
  (thyme and basil)
2 mild chiles, split in half (optional)
2 bay leaves
1 tablespoon peppercorns

TO MAKE ON THE STOVETOP

Place the vegetables, herbs, and seasoning into an 8-quart stockpot and fill with cold water, up to 1 inch below the top of the pot. Bring to a low simmer and let cook for a minimum of 90 minutes.

TO MAKE IN A CROCKPOT

Place the vegetables, herbs, and seasoning into a large crockpot and fill with cold water. Set heat to low and let cook for 4 hours.

When stock is finished cooking, strain it. Wait to add salt and other seasoning until you are ready to use the stock.

CHICKEN STOCK

You can simply add a small chicken to the vegetable stock base and increase the stovetop cook time to 3 hours (6–8 hours in a crockpot) to make homemade chicken stock. Personally, I find purchased chicken broth to consistently taste better than the beef or vegetable varieties. So if I'm taking the time to make homemade stock, I prefer to make beef or vegetable stock.

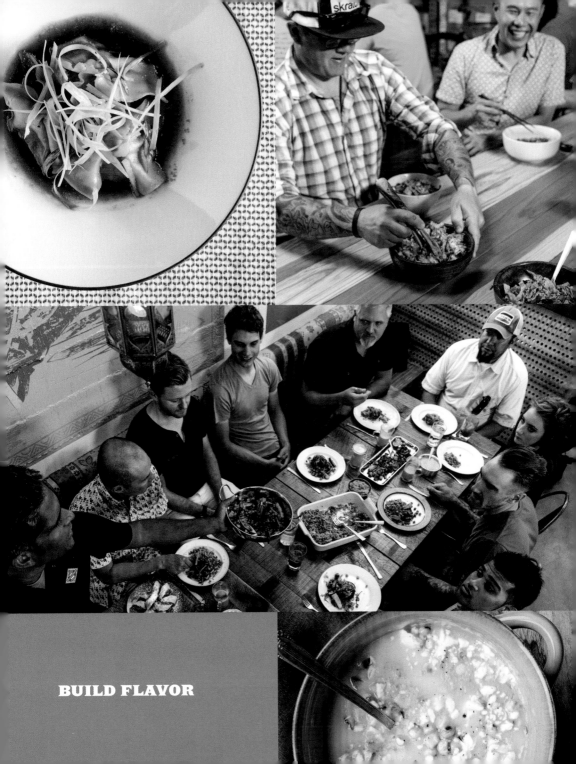

BUILD FLAVOR

CHILLED BLACK BEAN YOGURT SOUP

This is a pretty soup that takes very little time to make. The sour notes from the yogurt are the perfect setup for a hearty family meal. **Serves 6**

1 15-ounce can black beans
   or 2 cups cooked beans
½ cup diced red bell pepper
½ cup peeled and diced
   cucumber
2 tablespoons minced
   red onion
juice from half a lemon
1 teaspoon salt
1 quart plain yogurt
   (not Greek-style)

ON TOP
extra-virgin olive oil to drizzle
fresh lemon juice
1–2 hot peppers, chopped
   (optional)
¼ cup chopped fresh dill,
   fresh basil, or fresh parsley
   (optional)

If using canned beans, drain and rinse them. Put the beans, red bell pepper, cucumber, and red onion into a medium-sized mixing bowl and toss with lemon juice and salt. Reserve ¼ cup of the mixture for garnish.

Gently fold the yogurt into the bean mixture in the mixing bowl, being careful not to crush the beans. Finish with a drizzle of olive oil and a fresh squeeze of lemon, and garnish with the reserved black bean mixture along with spicy peppers and fresh herbs, if using.

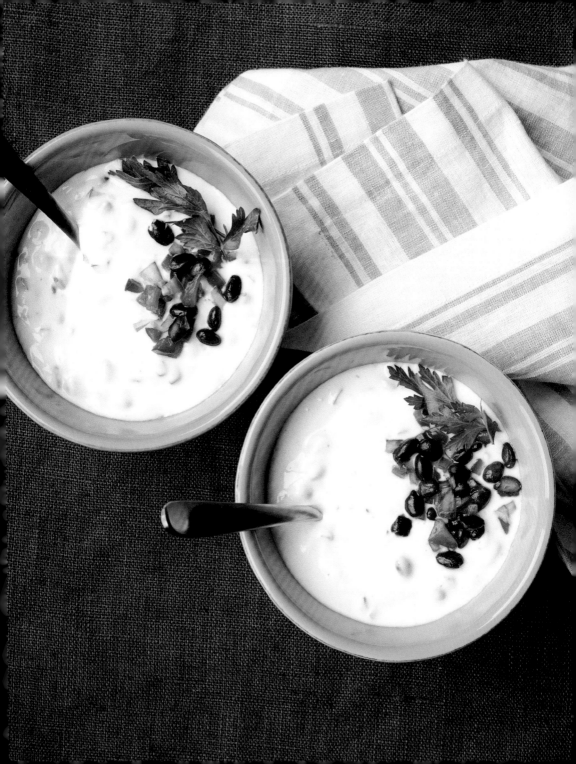

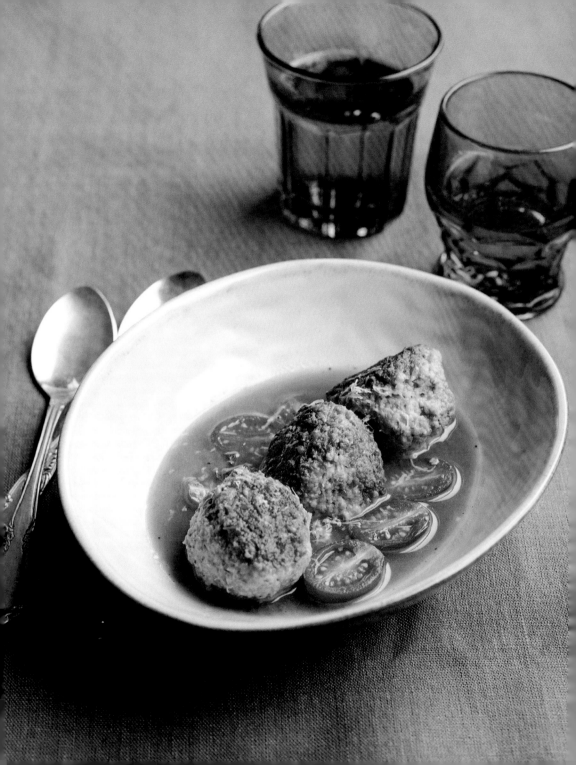

TURKEY MEATBALL & TOMATO SOUP

Turkey is more affordable than beef, and it has a nice, mild flavor. This is a versatile dish because it's really just meatballs in a tomato broth—a light but filling soup. Add grilled vegetables and serve it over cooked pasta or grains to make a bigger plate. **Serves 4**

1 pound ground turkey
2 cups gluten-free bread
  crumbs
2 tablespoons Italian seasoning
2 eggs, lightly beaten
1 teaspoon salt
⅛ teaspoon ground nutmeg
1 tablespoon olive oil
4 cups chicken stock
1 pint cherry or grape
  tomatoes, halved
2 tablespoons freshly
  grated Parmesan
salt and pepper to taste

In a large bowl, combine the ground turkey, bread crumbs, Italian seasoning, eggs, salt, and nutmeg. Work the mixture with your hands until well combined. Divide into 12 large meatballs, about the size of golf balls.

Heat a large sauté pan over medium heat, add the olive oil, and cook the meatballs for 10–15 minutes. Be careful not to crowd the pan or rush the process by turning up the heat. If the meatballs begin to stick to the pan, add a bit more olive oil. Use tongs to turn the meatballs until they have good color all around.

Add the chicken stock and tomatoes and cover the pan to bring it to a rolling boil. Cook the meatballs for another 5–10 minutes. Season to taste with freshly grated Parmesan and salt and pepper.

TORN BREAD & RADICCHIO SALAD

This free-form, rustic salad highlights some unique flavors and textures—bitter and peppery radicchio, sweet charred broccoli, and toasted bread and nuts to bring it all into balance. Keep in mind that once the salad is dressed, it doesn't keep so well, but you'll likely have some requests for seconds. **Serves 6**

half a loaf of rustic bread
3 tablespoons extra-virgin
   olive oil, divided
salt and pepper to taste
12 ounces broccoli florets
   (about 4–5 cups)
½ cup water
½ cup pine nuts or walnuts
1 small head radicchio, chopped
   into bite-sized chunks
2 tablespoons balsamic vinegar
juice from 1 lemon
2 tablespoons freshly
   grated Parmesan

Heat the oven to 350 degrees. Coarsely tear the bread into large chunks and place on a baking sheet. Brush with 1 tablespoon olive oil and season with salt and pepper. Place in the oven to bake for 10–15 minutes, or until the outer edges are toasted.

While the bread is toasting, steam the broccoli florets in ½ cup water in a shallow sauté pan over high heat with the lid on. Remove the lid to let the water evaporate from the pan and turn the heat up to high. Add 1 tablespoon olive oil and nuts. Cook long enough to crisp up the florets and toast the nuts. Remove from heat.

Combine the toasted bread and radicchio with the warm broccoli and pine nuts just before serving.

In a small bowl or measuring cup whisk together the remaining 1 tablespoon of olive oil, balsamic vinegar, and lemon juice.

Pour the dressing over the salad and toss to coat. Top with freshly grated Parmesan and season with salt and pepper to taste.

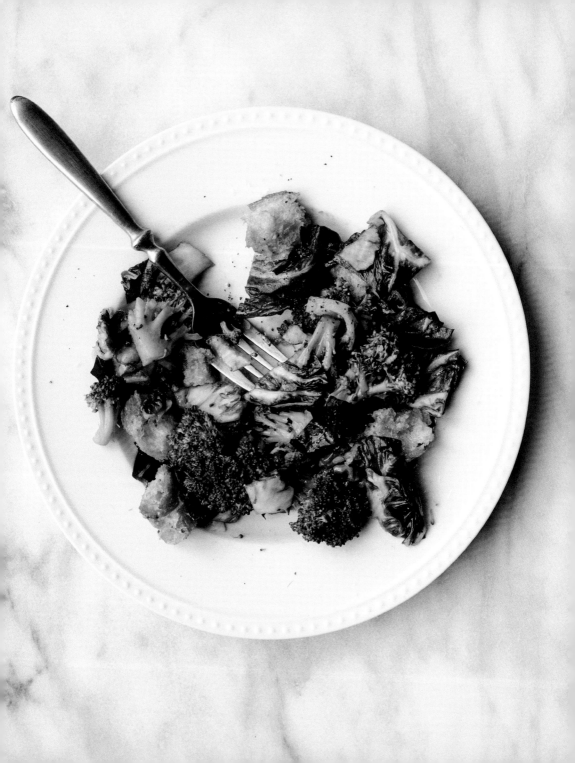

CHILE & LIME-SPICED BAY SCALLOPS

This is a super simple and fast way to make a bright and flavorful side. To serve this as an entrée, you can put it on top of cooked pasta. • Tiny bay scallops are usually affordable and easy to find at the grocery store. Large scallops work as well—just double the cooking time. **Serves 6**

1 pound bay scallops
¼ cup rice flour mixed with
   1 teaspoon Vindaloo Spice
   Mix (see p. 209) or 1
   teaspoon salt and ½
   teaspoon pepper
1 tablespoon coconut oil,
   divided
2 tablespoons chopped
   green onions
2 tablespoons chopped
   fresh cilantro
sprinkle of dry red chile
   or red pepper flakes
juice from 1 lime
chopped fresh chives

Begin by trimming the "foot," or tough tissue, off of the side of the scallops. (This is more prominent if you are working with larger scallops.) Rinse scallops and gently pat dry with paper towels. Lightly dust the scallops in the rice flour mixture on all sides.

Heat a sauté pan over high heat, adding just enough coconut oil to coat the bottom. Gently sear the scallops for approximately 2 minutes, or until golden brown. Use tongs to carefully flip them over, and cook the second side for another 1–2 minutes, or until the scallops are white in the center. Remove from heat and set aside.

In a small mixing bowl, combine the green onions, cilantro, and dry red chile or red pepper flakes. Add this mixture and the remaining coconut oil to the pan and stir gently.

Plate the scallops and finish with fresh-squeezed lime juice and fresh chives.

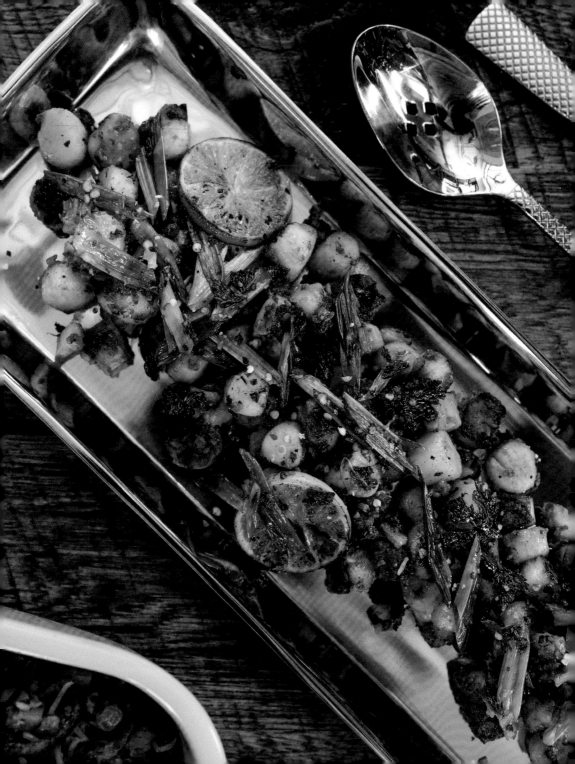

OLIVE OIL-POACHED TOMATO SOUP WITH WALNUTS

Fresh ripe tomatoes and a high-quality olive oil make this soup simple yet elegant. It's a great soup on a summer evening, with its warm amber notes. **Serves 4**

¼ cup olive oil
2 pounds tomatoes,
   quartered (about 8 cups)
½ teaspoon salt
½ cup walnuts or pecans
¼ cup torn fresh basil leaves
juice from 1 lemon
salt and pepper to taste
drizzle of extra-virgin olive oil
   or balsamic vinegar

Heat a medium pot over medium-high heat and warm the olive oil. Add the quartered tomatoes and salt and cook for about 10 minutes, or until the color begins to darken.

While the tomatoes are cooking, toast the nuts in a dry pan over medium-high heat. Use a wooden spoon to stir frequently. Once the nuts turn golden, remove from heat and set aside to cool.

Transfer the poached tomatoes and olive oil to a blender. Pulse to purée.

Season the soup to taste with the torn basil leaves, lemon juice, and salt and pepper. Serve in individual bowls with a drizzle of olive oil or balsamic vinegar and a small handful of toasted nuts.

PAIRS WELL WITH PEPPER-CRUSTED COD (P. 196) OR GRILLED CHEESE, NATURALLY.

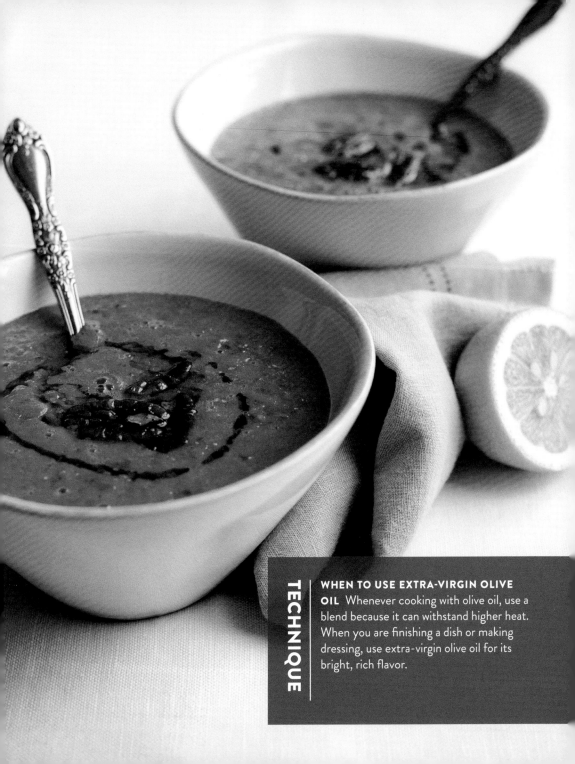

TECHNIQUE

WHEN TO USE EXTRA-VIRGIN OLIVE OIL Whenever cooking with olive oil, use a blend because it can withstand higher heat. When you are finishing a dish or making dressing, use extra-virgin olive oil for its bright, rich flavor.

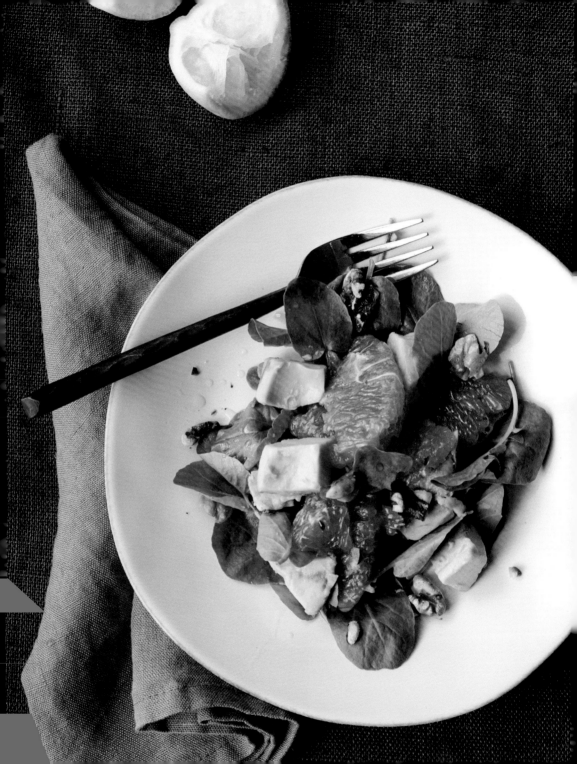

FRESH GRAPEFRUIT & AVOCADO SALAD

This is the perfect light salad for summertime. Dense, rich avocado pairs beautifully with bitter greens and fresh grapefruit. Put together each plate separately to keep the grapefruit intact and impress your friends with this delicate salad. **Serves 6**

½ cup walnuts
2 large grapefruits
2 cups fresh watercress or
    other bitter greens such
    as arugula or chard
2 firm ripe avocados, cut into
    large bite-sized pieces
2 tablespoons extra-virgin
    olive oil
juice from 1 lemon
2 teaspoons honey
salt and pepper to taste

Gently toast the walnuts in a dry sauté pan until they warm up and become fragrant.
Set aside to cool.

To prepare the grapefruit, first peel off the skin by hand. Gently pull apart each section, removing all of the white bits (pith and membrane) while keeping the fruit intact.

Layer each plate with watercress or other greens, then add the grapefruit, followed by avocado and walnuts.

In a small bowl whisk together the olive oil, lemon juice, and honey for the dressing.

Top each salad with a splash of dressing and salt and freshly ground pepper to taste. Depending on how bitter your grapefruit is, you might want more salt.

THIS MAKES A BRIGHT ACCOMPANIMENT TO THE BAKED SALMON IN PASTRY (P. 191).

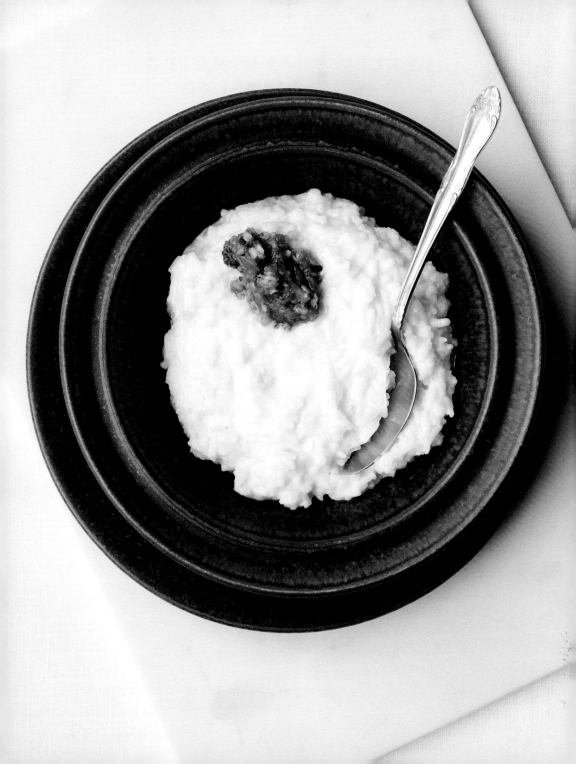

COCONUT RICE PORRIDGE
WITH ADACHERRI

Adacherri is a spicy, fresh ground chutney popular in South India. In my home growing up, it could accompany just about any dish, at any time of the day. Here we use it to heat up this simple rice porridge. • Look for tamarind pulp at the Asian market. You can also substitute balsamic vinegar; just reduce the quantity to keep the color bright. **Serves 4**

2 cups leftover rice
   (nonsticky is best for this)
1 cup coconut milk
2 tablespoons warm water
½ teaspoon salt

ADACHERRI
1 cup coarsely chopped
   fresh chiles (serrano,
   jalapeño, Thai)
2 tablespoons coarsely
   chopped fresh shallot
1 teaspoon minced fresh ginger
a few sprigs of fresh cilantro
2 cloves garlic, smashed
1 tablespoon tamarind pulp or
   1 teaspoon balsamic vinegar
1 tablespoon coconut oil,
   melted
1 teaspoon salt
juice from 1 lime
8–10 fresh curry leaves
   (optional)

If you don't have leftover rice on hand, combine 1 cup of rice, 1½ cups water, and a dash of salt in a rice cooker or cook the rice on the stovetop.

TO MAKE THE ADACHERRI: Put all of the ingredients in a food processor and pulse until incorporated. Taste, and if the sauce is too spicy, add a bit more coconut oil. The sauce will keep in the refrigerator for up to 1 week. Makes about 1 cup.

TO MAKE THE PORRIDGE: In a saucepan over medium-high heat, bring the cooked rice, coconut milk, warm water, and salt to a low simmer. As the pot warms, the rice will begin to absorb the liquid and the mixture will thicken.

Ladle into individual bowls and serve with a dollop of adacherri.

PAIRS WELL WITH RUSTIC CHICKEN (P. 140).

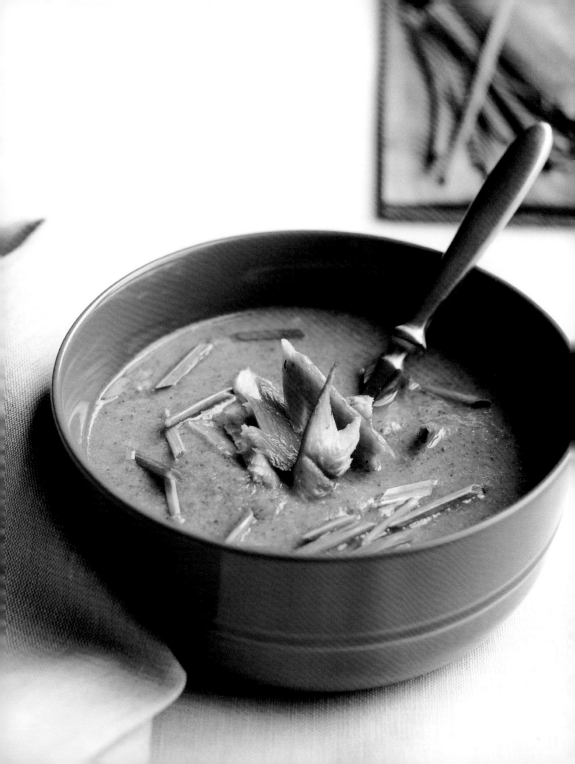

BROCCOLI SOUP WITH
SMOKED TROUT & CHIVES

Delicious hot or cold, this is a soup that you can enjoy throughout the year. You'll be amazed at how good a few simple ingredients can taste. Dress it up with smoked trout and chives, and you'll be happy to get your fill of broccoli. **Serves 6**

2 pounds broccoli crowns
½ cup minced onion
8 cups water
2 teaspoons salt
juice from half a lemon
salt and pepper to taste

ON TOP
3–4 ounces smoked trout filet,
   flaked
¼ cup chopped fresh chives
freshly grated Parmesan
   (optional)

In a large pot over medium-high heat, simmer the broccoli and onion in salted water until just tender, about 8–10 minutes. The color should still be vibrant.

Transfer the cooked broccoli, onions, and liquid to a blender or a food processor and purée in batches until the soup reaches a smooth consistency. Season to taste with a squeeze of lemon, salt, and pepper.

Return the soup to the pan to bring back to heat before serving. Serve in individual bowls topped with smoked trout, fresh chives, and Parmesan. If you are not using the trout, a splash of good extra-virgin olive oil can finish off the soup nicely.

SPICY RED BEANS & RICE

If you are cooking for kids, this is the kind of comfort food that they crave. To keep the dish mild, just reserve the red pepper flakes and jalapeño for garnishing individual bowls and everyone wins. • Adzuki or kidney beans work well in this recipe. **Serves 6**

1 cup (6 ounces) minced bacon
12 ounces smoked sausage, diced
1 cup minced onions
1 cup minced celery
4 cloves garlic, minced
1 tablespoon red pepper flakes
2 cups uncooked medium-grain white rice (jasmine)
1 tablespoon Creole seasoning
1 14.5-ounce can crushed or diced tomatoes, or about 2 cups chopped fresh tomatoes
2 cups water or stock
1 15-ounce can red beans or 2 cups cooked red beans
2 tablespoons minced jalapeño

ON TOP
Tabasco (optional)
plain yogurt (optional)

Begin by browning the bacon and sausage in a deep skillet over medium-high heat. Drain off any excess fat, then add onions, celery, garlic, and red pepper flakes and cook until the onions are translucent.

Add uncooked rice and Creole seasoning while scraping the bottom of the pan. Once the mixture is evenly combined, reduce heat to medium and add tomatoes and water or stock. Cover and cook for approximately 15–20 minutes, or until most of the liquid is absorbed.

If using canned beans, drain and rinse them, then add red beans and jalapeño to the skillet. Continue to cook another 5 minutes, or until the rice is tender. The mixture may stick to the bottom of the pan, so be careful to keep scraping and moving it all around.

Serve with a splash of Tabasco and a dollop of plain yogurt.

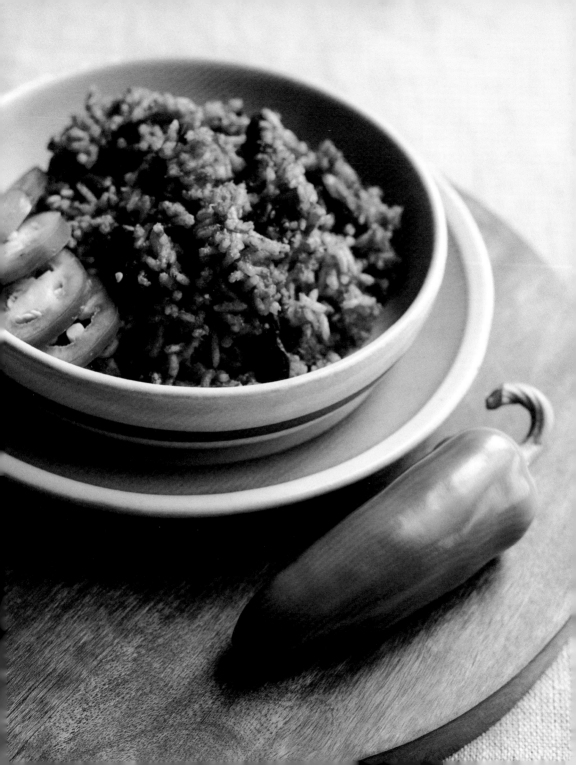

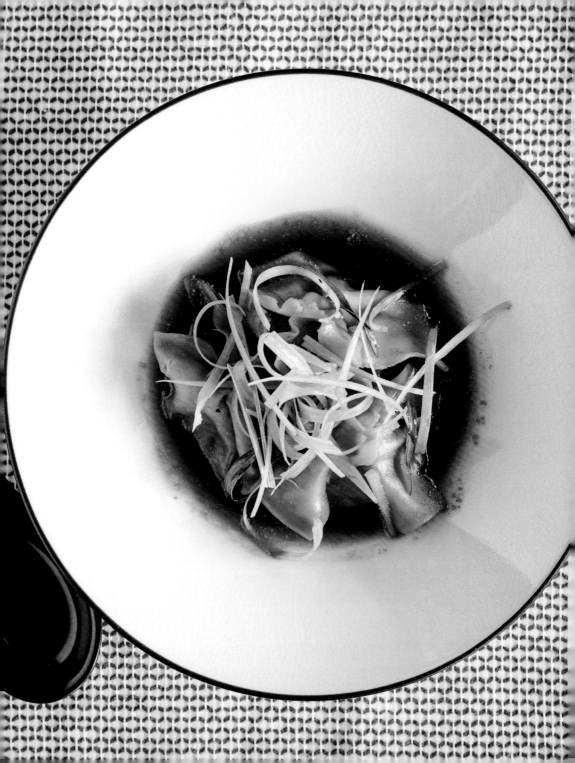

SWEET POTATO-STUFFED WONTON SOUP

Simple soups like this one are made amazing with homemade stock, but the recipe that follows includes enough flavor to work well with a store-bought stock too. Because these varieties typically contain more sodium, be sure to add the soy sauce or red miso paste incrementally, tasting as you go, so it doesn't get too salty. **Serves 6**

1 pound sweet potatoes, peeled and diced (about 3 cups)
1 cup chopped pecans
¼ teaspoon nutmeg
½ teaspoon salt
1 packet (about 3 dozen) wonton wrappers, round or small squares

SOY GINGER BROTH
4 cups beef or vegetable stock
½ cup low-sodium soy sauce or red miso paste
2 garlic cloves, minced
1 thumb fresh ginger, peeled and sliced into thin matchsticks
½ teaspoon whole peppercorns
salt to taste

ON TOP
¼ cup thinly sliced green onions
fresh tarragon (optional)

TO MAKE THE FILLING: Bring a large pot of salted water to a rolling boil and add sweet potatoes. Cook 12–15 minutes, or until soft enough to mash. Drain the potatoes—if they are not well drained, the filling will be soupy.

Transfer the sweet potatoes into a medium bowl and mash with a sturdy wire whisk or a fork. Add the pecans, nutmeg, and salt and mash together.

TO MAKE THE WONTONS: Brush lukewarm water along the edge of each wonton skin and add 1 teaspoon of filling. Bring all four corners up to the top and seal the edges to form a square pocket. This recipe makes about 36 dumplings.

TO MAKE THE SOY GINGER BROTH: In a large pot over medium-high heat combine the stock and soy sauce or red miso paste. Taste the soy sauce or miso for salt before adding and adjust the quantity as needed. Add garlic, ginger, and peppercorns and bring to a low rolling boil.

Drop the wontons into the broth and cook until they float, approximately 5 minutes.

Serve in individual bowls, ladling 6 dumplings into each one. Season with salt to taste and garnish with green onions and fresh tarragon, if using.

Note: You can freeze any leftover filling or wonton skins for next time.

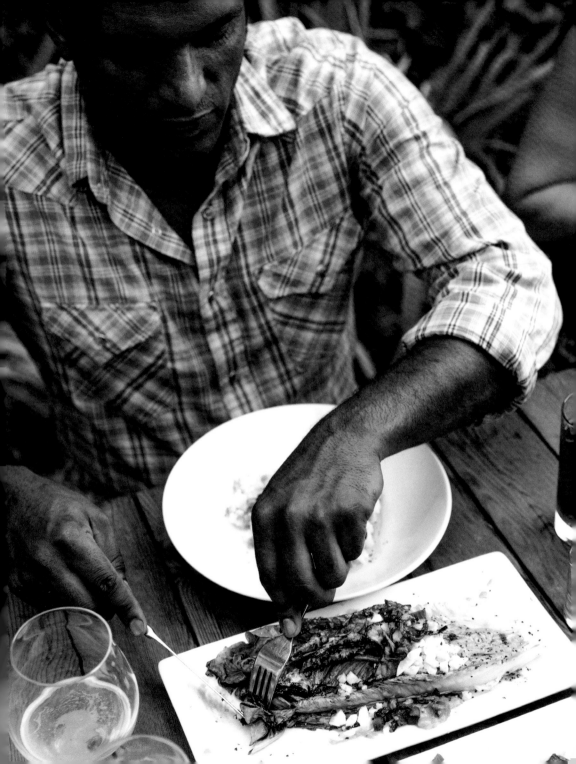

GRILLED ROMAINE WITH PANCETTA, HARD-BOILED EGGS & DIJON DRESSING

A little time on the grill elevates romaine lettuce from everyday to gourmet. As a chef, I love to char hearty greens for a slightly bitter, smoky flavor that pairs beautifully with corn and pancetta. This salad is one of the first things I showed Allen how to bust out on his trusty Weber. Get all the toppings prepped and chopped, and they can wait in the fridge. Grill the romaine just before dinner and from there it's easy assembly. **Serves 6**

4 eggs
2 ears fresh sweet corn,
    kernels cut off the cob
8 ounces thick-cut pancetta
    or bacon, chopped
1 cup thinly sliced onion
3 hearts of romaine
olive oil
coarse salt and pepper to taste

DIJON DRESSING
¼ cup extra-virgin olive oil
1 tablespoon Dijon mustard
juice from half a lemon
¼ teaspoon coarse salt

TO PREPARE THE TOPPINGS: Bring a pot of water to a low rolling boil, and carefully add the eggs. Cook for 12 minutes, then remove from heat and immediately run under cold water while cracking the shells slightly. Let rest in cold water for a few minutes—this should make it much easier to remove the peel.

While the eggs are cooking, place the corn in a dry sauté pan over medium-high heat and cook until lightly charred. Remove from pan and set aside.

In the same pan, cook the pancetta or bacon over medium heat until crispy. Transfer the pancetta or bacon to a plate lined with a paper towel, drain the bulk of the grease, and use the same pan to sauté the onion until the edges become crisp and lightly browned.

Once the eggs are cool to the touch, drain the water and peel away the shell. Chop coarsely.

TO MAKE THE DRESSING: In a small bowl, whisk together the ingredients for the dressing.

(recipe continues)

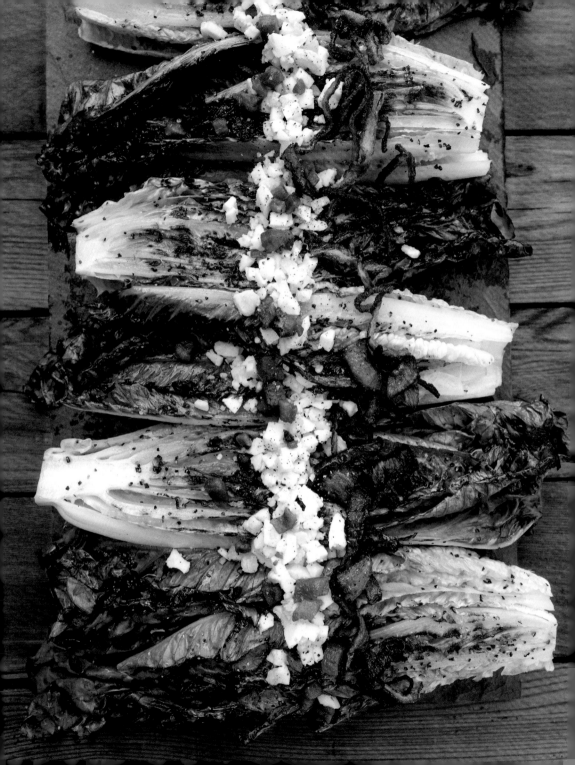

TO GRILL THE LETTUCE: Bring the grill or grill pan to medium-high heat. Slice the romaine in half lengthwise and lightly brush with olive oil. Grill the romaine cut-side down until you get some crisp, charred edges, about 5–6 minutes. Use tongs to carefully jiggle and release the romaine if preparing on the grill, and arrange it on a large serving platter.

Generously sprinkle the grilled lettuce with all of the toppings: hard-boiled eggs, corn, pancetta or bacon, and onions.

Finish with coarse salt and pepper and a generous drizzle of Dijon dressing.

SERVE THIS SALAD AS AN ENTRÉE WITH PASTA WITH MAPLE CARROTS & LEEKS (P. 135) ON THE SIDE.

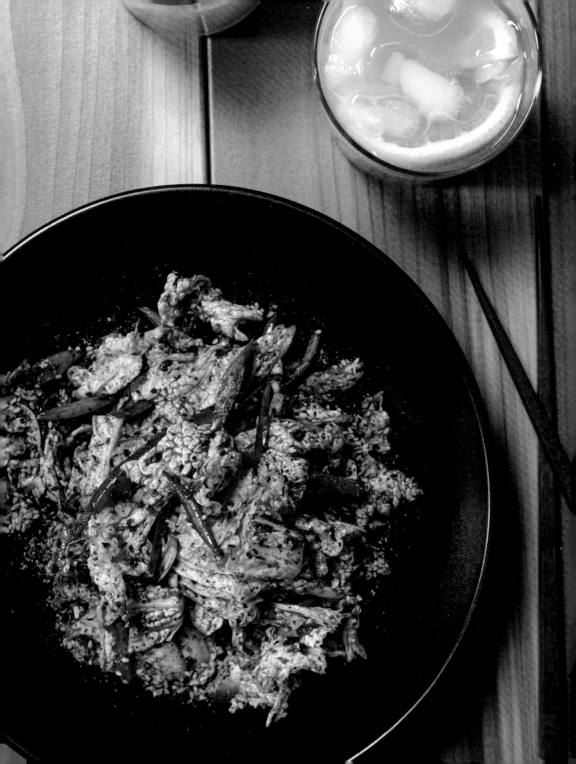

KIMCHEE
SPICED SALAD

The bold flavors of kimchee can be used to make a light, flavorful salad that works amazingly well as a base for your favorite proteins, such as grilled tofu or chicken. This salad is also pretty fantastic with an over-easy egg and rice. The secret is Korean red pepper, which you can find at the Asian market. It is surprisingly mild with a silky, toasted texture that almost melts in your mouth. **Serves 4**

1 napa cabbage or bok choy,
    thinly sliced
1 bunch green onions,
    thinly sliced
1 jalapeño, thinly sliced
1 tablespoon toasted
    sesame seeds
juice from half a lemon

**RED PEPPER SESAME OIL
DRESSING**
½ cup spicy Korean red pepper
    (you can add a lot more
    if you'd like)
¼ cup rice wine vinegar
¼ cup sesame oil
1 teaspoon coarse salt
juice from 1 lemon,
    plus additional to taste

Combine the napa cabbage or bok choy with green onions, jalapeño, and sesame seeds in a large bowl. Toss with a squeeze of lemon juice to soften the cabbage and set aside while you make the dressing.

TO MAKE THE DRESSING: In a separate bowl, combine the Korean red pepper, vinegar, sesame oil, and salt. Whisk in the lemon juice. You can also add a splash of cold water to thin the paste. Adjust to taste with additional lemon juice or water.

Add the dressing to the cabbage mixture and toss until evenly distributed. Serve right away.

Note: If you can't find Korean red pepper, combine 1 cup sweet paprika and ¼ cup mild red pepper flakes in a dry pan and warm over medium heat, stirring consistently for 2–4 minutes until slightly toasted, but not smoking.

SHOWN WITH SPARKING GINGER SODA (P. 64).

CITRUS SALAD WITH YUZU DRESSING & WONTON CRISPS

Yuzu is a Japanese citrus with a delightfully strong flavor reminiscent of creamy vanilla and lemon flowers. Just a splash is all you need. While it's particularly nice on this salad, yuzu can be hard to find and a little expensive, so citrus makes a good substitute. This dressing can also be used to finish stir-fried vegetables or rice. The salad goes particularly well with pork or Asian-inspired dishes. **Serves 6**

¼ cup vegetable oil
8 wonton skins, cut into strips
1 head lettuce
¼ head red cabbage,
   thinly sliced
2 oranges
1 tablespoon toasted
   sesame seeds

YUZU DRESSING

¼ cup yuzu juice or juice from
   1 lemon and half an orange
1 tablespoon white miso paste
1 teaspoon water
2 tablespoons sesame oil
½ teaspoon coarse sugar
   or agave
salt and pepper to taste

TO MAKE WONTON CRISPS: Warm the vegetable oil in a small sauté pan over medium-high heat. Once the oil is hot, carefully add the wonton strips and use tongs to flip them after a few minutes. Once they are a crispy golden brown, drain the wonton crisps on a plate lined with a paper towel and set aside to cool. Wonton crisps can be stored in an airtight container for several days.

TO MAKE THE SALAD: Pull apart the lettuce, tear into bite-sized pieces, and place in a large mixing bowl. Add the cabbage. Peel the oranges and cut them up into large pieces. Set aside.

TO MAKE THE DRESSING: Whisk together the ingredients for the dressing and season to taste with salt and pepper. Toss with the lettuce and cabbage and top with orange sections, wonton crisps, and toasted sesame seeds.

A GREAT SIDE SALAD WITH COUNTRY-STYLE HOISIN RIBS (P. 219).

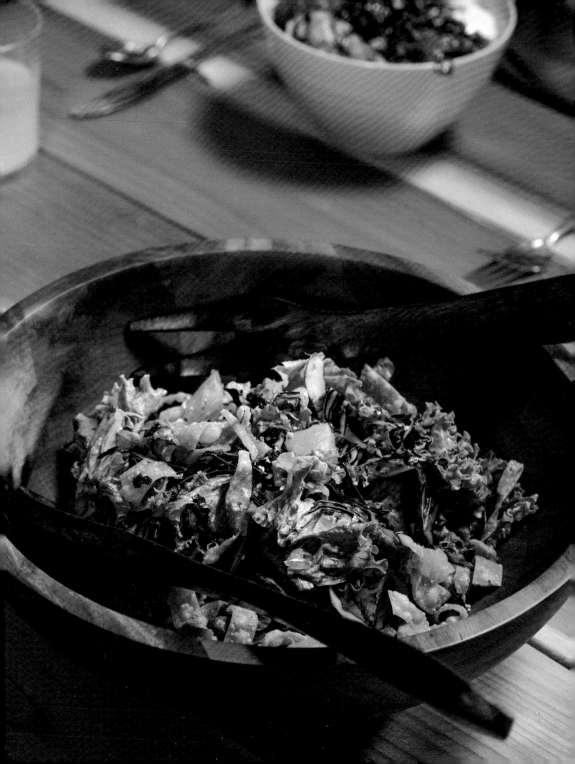

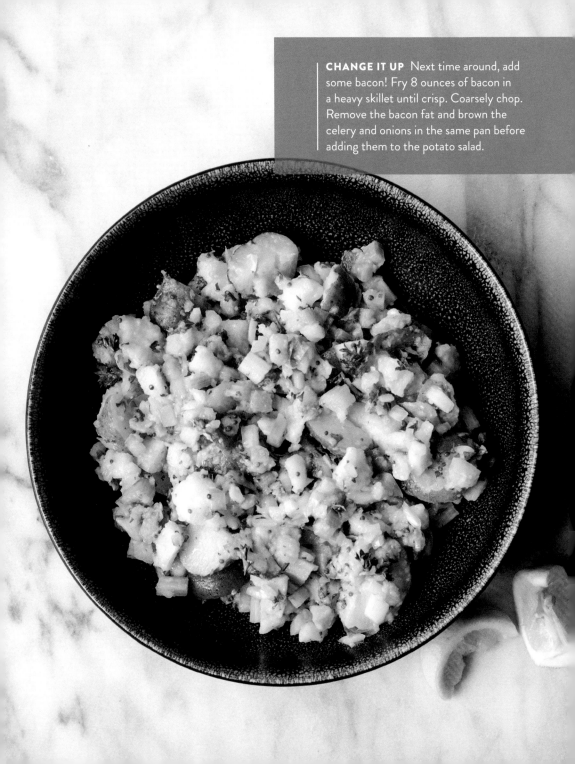

CHANGE IT UP Next time around, add some bacon! Fry 8 ounces of bacon in a heavy skillet until crisp. Coarsely chop. Remove the bacon fat and brown the celery and onions in the same pan before adding them to the potato salad.

WARM GERMAN POTATO SALAD

Gently smashed potatoes play well as a side or as the base for just about any protein. We typically associate potato salads with summertime grilling, but a warm potato salad like this one belongs on the table with hearty meals in the fall and winter months, too. **Serves 4**

1 pound small red potatoes, quartered (about 3 cups)
¼ cup white vinegar
¼ cup extra-virgin olive oil
1 tablespoon coarse-ground mustard
1 cup minced celery and celery leaves
¼ cup minced onion
¼ cup chopped fresh parsley
½ teaspoon coarse salt
¼ teaspoon pepper
¼ teaspoon coarse sugar
additional salt and pepper to taste
juice from half a lemon

Bring a large pot of salted water to a rolling boil and add the potatoes. Once the water returns to a boil, cook for 12–15 minutes, or until the potatoes are fork tender. Drain the potatoes and set aside to cool for a moment.

While the potatoes are cooking, mix the dressing. In a large measuring cup, whisk together the vinegar, olive oil, and mustard.

Place the celery, onion, and parsley in a mixing bowl. Add the potatoes while they are still warm and gently mash them with the other ingredients. Pour the dressing over the potato mixture and add in coarse salt, pepper, and sugar.

Adjust flavor with additional salt and pepper as needed, finish with a squeeze of lemon, and serve warm.

PAN-ROASTED CHICKPEAS & SUMMER VEGETABLES

This side dish combines great textures and colors that work well with most any entrée. Use whatever seasonal vegetables you can get in place of squash—broccoli florets, Brussels sprouts, small tomatoes, spring peas, or fresh sweet corn. **Serves 6**

1 15-ounce can chickpeas or
   2 cups cooked chickpeas
6 medium yellow and
   green squash
   (about 3 pounds)
2 tablespoons coconut oil,
   divided
salt and pepper to taste
½ teaspoon ground cinnamon
¼ cup coarsely chopped
   fresh basil
¼ cup coarsely chopped
   fresh cilantro
½ cup crumbled feta or other
   fresh sheep's milk cheese
   (optional)

In a strainer, drain and rinse the chickpeas and let dry for a few minutes while cutting the vegetables.

Quarter the squash lengthwise and chop into 2-inch pieces. Any thick cut will work—the squash is less likely to overcook this way.

Once the chickpeas are dry, add 1 tablespoon of coconut oil to a sauté pan and cook them over medium-high heat until crisp. Dust with salt, pepper, and ground cinnamon, and set aside.

Panfry the squash (or other vegetables) in the remaining coconut oil in small batches. Combine with the toasted chickpeas and sprinkle with chopped herbs and feta (if using) before serving.

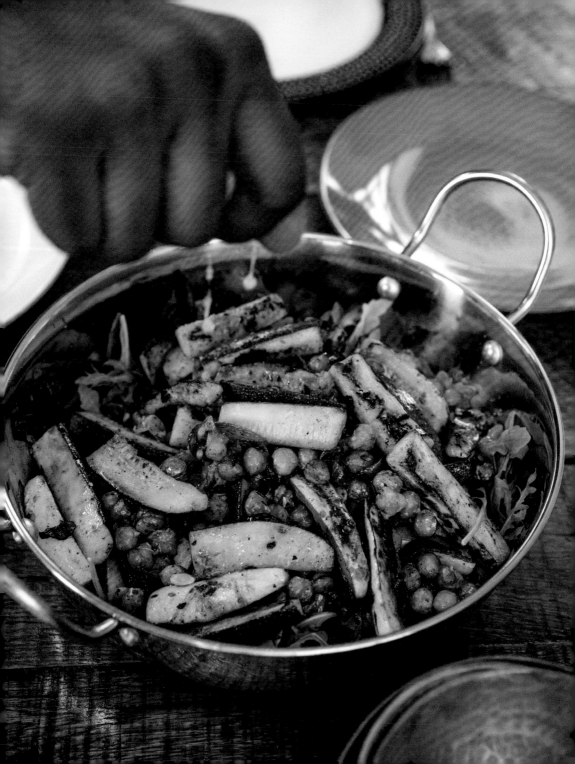

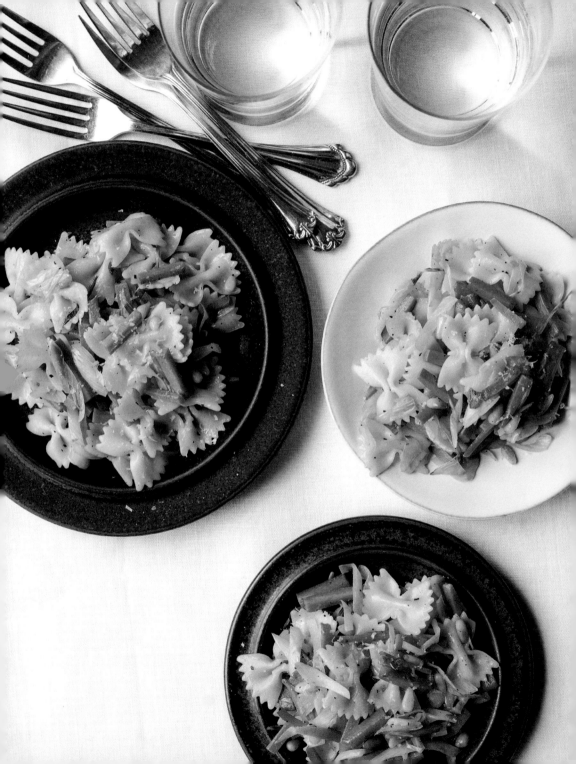

PASTA WITH
MAPLE CARROTS & LEEKS

This dish is quick to prepare, whether you are looking for a light lunch or a last-minute side dish. With a hint of sweetness and toasted pine nuts, it makes a great companion for holiday fare—turkey or roasted meats. **Serves 4**

8 ounces uncooked
  farfalle pasta
2 tablespoons olive oil
4 carrots, cut into small
  matchsticks
2 cups thinly sliced leeks,
  including tender green parts
½ cup pine nuts
½ cup vegetable stock
2 tablespoons maple syrup
1 handful of fresh herbs
  (parsley or tarragon)
coarse salt and pepper to taste
1 teaspoon crushed red pepper
freshly grated Parmesan
  (optional)

Bring a large pot of salted water to a boil and prepare the pasta as directed on the package. Drain and set aside.

Warm the olive oil in a sauté pan over medium-high heat. Add the carrots, leeks, and pine nuts and cook until the carrots become tender and the pine nuts turn a golden brown, about 5 minutes. Add the stock and cook just long enough to bring to a low simmer.

Remove from heat and stir in the maple syrup. Add the cooked pasta and toss with fresh herbs. Finish with salt and pepper to taste and top with crushed red pepper and Parmesan, if desired.

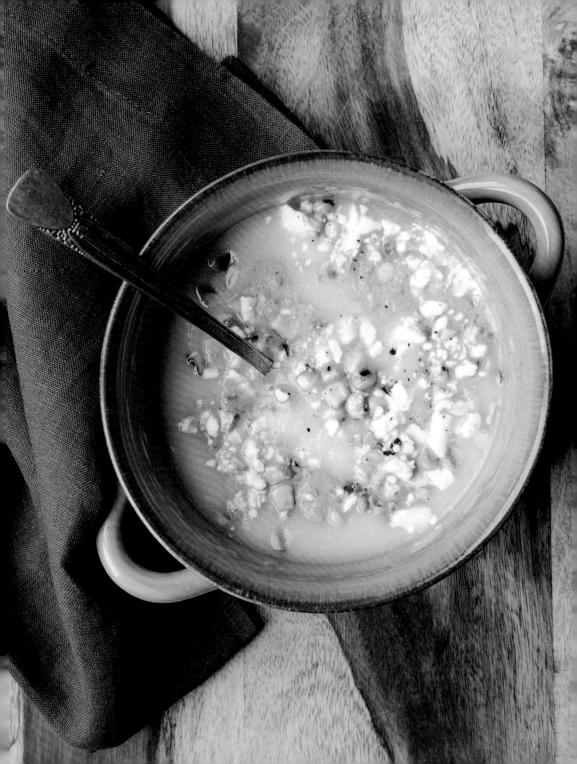

CAULIFLOWER & CORN CHOWDER WITH RED PEPPER OIL

This is a light soup that pairs well with a hearty chopped salad or roasted chicken. Be sure to use all of the cauliflower, stalk included. **Serves 6**

1 quart chicken stock
1 pound cauliflower (1 large head), coarsely chopped
2 ears fresh sweet corn, cut off the cob (or 2 cups frozen corn), divided
1 cup plain yogurt, divided

RED PEPPER OIL
1 red bell pepper
2 tablespoons extra-virgin olive oil
coarse salt to taste

ON TOP
2 tablespoons farmer or feta cheese, crumbled
1 tablespoon chopped fresh parsley or basil (optional)
coarsely ground black pepper to taste

TO MAKE THE RED PEPPER OIL: Blanch the bell pepper in salted boiling water for no more than 1 minute. The skin will be wrinkled. Run the pepper under cold water, then peel off the skin and remove the stem and seeds. Place the pepper in a blender with the olive oil and purée. Season to taste with coarse salt and set aside.

TO MAKE THE CHOWDER: In a large pot over medium-high heat, bring the chicken stock to a rolling boil and simmer the cauliflower for about 10 minutes, or until fork tender.

While the cauliflower is cooking, char the corn in a dry sauté pan over medium-high heat, stirring to keep it from blackening. Set aside.

Transfer the cooked cauliflower and chicken stock into a food processor and purée until smooth. Return the cauliflower mixture to the pot and fold in half the corn and half the yogurt. Cook for another minute or two over low heat to warm throughout.

Pour chowder into individual bowls and top with remaining corn, a spoonful of yogurt, and a drizzle of red pepper oil. Garnish with fresh crumbled cheese and fresh chopped herbs, if using. Finish with coarsely ground black pepper.

THE GO-TO MEAT

*When choosing what meat to serve to your guests,
chicken is typically the safest choice.
It's the smallest offender, both to your budget and the
environment, while still delivering plenty of taste.*

CHICKEN

RUSTIC
LEMON CHICKEN

This roasted chicken with flavors of lemon and garlic is surprisingly simple to make. You can also use a whole chicken. **Serves 6**

6 leg quarters, about 3 pounds
olive oil
5 garlic cloves, chopped
red pepper flakes to taste
coarse salt to taste
½ cup chopped fresh herbs
    (any combination of parsley,
    thyme, rosemary, and
    tarragon), divided
1 lemon, half of it sliced

Drizzle the chicken thoroughly with olive oil and then rub it with the chopped garlic, red pepper flakes, and salt. If you have the time, let the chicken rest at room temperature for up to 30 minutes. This isn't critical, but it makes for better flavor.

Adjust oven rack to the middle position and heat the broiler to high. Place the chicken skin-side up in a roasting pan. Top with half of the fresh chopped herbs (reserve the rest for garnish) and a few slices of lemon. Transfer the pan to the oven. Using the broiler will give the meat a nice color and texture, but it will create smoke, so make sure to vent your kitchen or turn the fan on. After 5–10 minutes you should have a nice, crisp, slightly charred finish.

Switch the oven from broil to bake and adjust the temperature to 375 degrees. Bake for 60 minutes, or until the meat reaches an internal temperature of 165 degrees.

Let the chicken cool for at least 10 minutes. Finish with the remaining fresh herbs and a squeeze of lemon before serving. Serve whole or chop apart the drumstick and thigh before serving.

TASTES GREAT WITH RADICCHIO SLAW (P. 246) AND KABOCHA SQUASH MASH (P. 204)

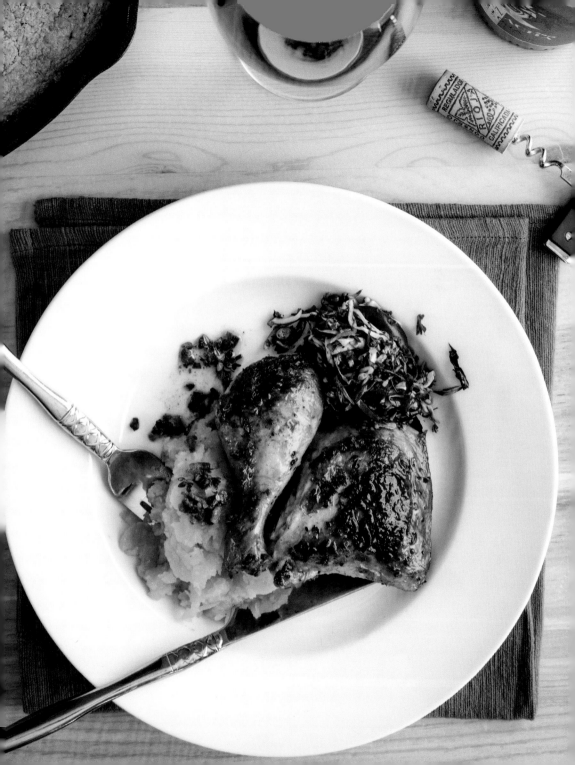

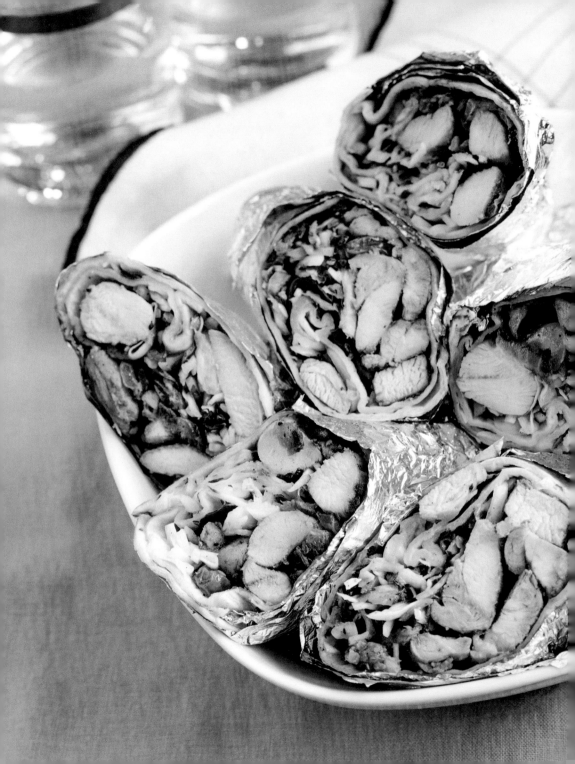

MASALA CHICKEN WRAP
WITH CABBAGE SLAW

This is an easy "make-ahead" recipe. You can also serve it as a chilled chicken salad. The cabbage slaw adds a little crunch, which is especially nice when you bite into a wrap. At the Little Curry Shop we use this slaw to finish off our rice dishes. Look for pliable tortillas or wraps that are at least 10 inches in diameter so you can pack in plenty of flavor. **Serves 6**

1 pound boneless, skinless
   chicken breasts
½ teaspoon salt
pepper to taste
1 tablespoon olive oil
¼ cup diced red onion
1 tablespoon curry powder
¼ cup raisins
1 cup plain yogurt
6 10-inch tortillas

CABBAGE SLAW
1 cup thinly sliced red cabbage
1 cup thinly sliced
   green cabbage
2 jalapeños, sliced into
   thin strips
½ cup cilantro leaves,
   loosely packed
¼ cup chopped green onions
   (optional)
¼ cup chopped radishes
   (optional)
½ teaspoon red pepper flakes
juice from 1 lemon
salt to taste
sprinkle of coarse sugar

Season the chicken with salt and pepper and cut into 1-inch cubes. Heat a sauté pan over medium-high heat, then add the olive oil. Add the cubed chicken and cook for 6–7 minutes, or until it begins to brown, stirring occasionally. Set the chicken aside to cool. (You can also grill the chicken. Leave the breasts whole and cook for 6–7 minutes on each side. Let cool before cutting into cubes.)

Use the same pan to sauté the diced onions over high heat. You can add a little oil if needed, but leaving the pan dry will give the onions a slightly charred texture. Once the onions begin to brown, stir in the curry powder and raisins and set aside.

In a large bowl combine the yogurt with the cooked onion and raisin mixture. Once the chicken has cooled, fold it into the yogurt mixture until it is thoroughly coated and refrigerate it while you make the slaw.

TO MAKE THE SLAW: Mix cabbage, jalapeños, cilantro, and any optional ingredients you are using in a medium-sized bowl. Right before serving, add the red pepper flakes, lemon juice, salt, and sugar. Toss to combine well.

To assemble, warm the tortillas one at a time in a warm, dry pan, being careful not to burn them. Load up each tortilla with the chicken and slaw, wrap like you would a burrito, and enjoy!

KALAMATA CHICKEN WITH NEW POTATOES

When I have friends coming over, this is one of my go-to dishes because I typically have these ingredients on hand. By starting the chicken on the stove and finishing it in the oven, all of these rustic flavors cook up nicely together. Serve piping hot over your favorite rice or grain. **Serves 6**

1½ pounds small potatoes (new red potatoes or Yukon gold), cut in half
4 skinless, boneless chicken breasts
½ cup all-purpose flour mixed with 1 teaspoon salt and ½ teaspoon pepper
2 tablespoons olive oil
1 large onion, diced large
6 garlic cloves, smashed
1 14.5-ounce can crushed tomatoes or 2 cups diced fresh tomatoes
1 cup pitted Kalamata olives
¼ cup coarsely chopped fresh parsley
¼ cup chopped fresh basil
salt and pepper to taste

Boil the potatoes in a large saucepan filled with salted water for about 15 minutes or until fork tender.

Meanwhile, cut each of the chicken breasts into 6 large pieces, first slicing each breast lengthwise, and then into thirds.

Heat the oven to 375 degrees.

Dust the chicken in the flour mixture and shake off excess. Heat an ovenproof sauté pan over medium-high heat, coat with olive oil, and panfry the chicken until it is lightly golden on all sides, approximately 8–10 minutes.

Drain the potatoes and set aside.

Add the onion and smashed garlic to the pan containing the chicken and cook a few more minutes, or until the onions are translucent. Add the cooked potatoes as well as the tomatoes, olives, and parsley and transfer the sauté pan to the middle rack of the oven to let the flavors come together as the dish finishes cooking, about 20 minutes.

Remove the pan from the oven and top with fresh basil, adding salt and pepper to taste.

ALSO SERVE WITH FRESH SPINACH PASTA (P. 152).

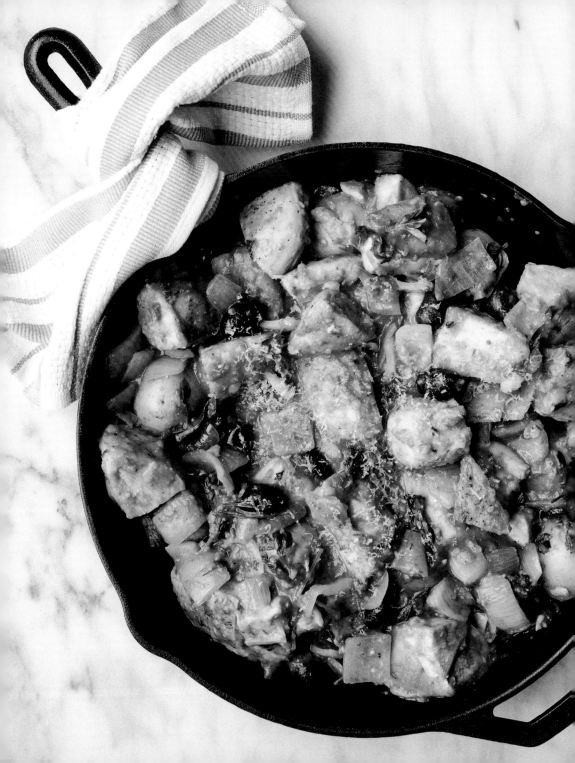

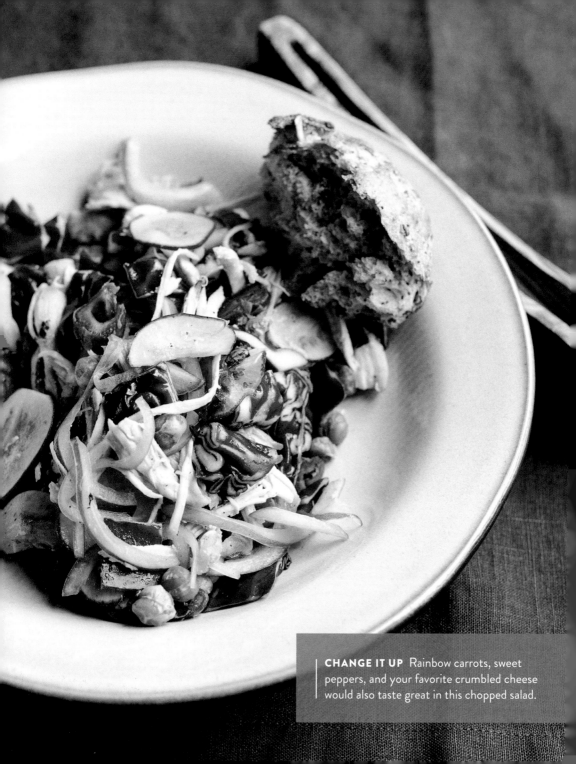

CHANGE IT UP Rainbow carrots, sweet peppers, and your favorite crumbled cheese would also taste great in this chopped salad.

CHOPPED CHICKEN SALAD WITH PICKLED ONIONS & RADISHES

This is a great last-minute salad to make use of leftover chicken. You can change it up throughout the year. The flash-pickled onions and radishes are the star of the dish. The combination of the vinegar, a touch of sugar, and salt balances out the strong flavors beautifully. **Serves 4**

2 cups shredded or chopped
   roasted chicken
salt and pepper to taste
1 cup canned or cooked
   chickpeas
1 teaspoon olive oil
½ head red cabbage,
   thinly sliced
¼ cup chopped dates, figs,
   or your favorite dried fruit
2 tablespoons coarsely
   chopped fresh cilantro
   or parsley, plus additional
   to finish
juice from 1 lemon
drizzle of maple syrup

PICKLED ONIONS & RADISHES

½ cup red onion,
   sliced into thin strips
4 radishes, sliced into
   thin rounds
¼ cup red wine vinegar
½ teaspoon coarse sugar
½ teaspoon coarse salt
¼ teaspoon crushed
   red pepper

TO MAKE THE PICKLED ONIONS: Combine the red onion and radishes with the red wine vinegar, coarse sugar and salt, and red pepper. Toss together and let sit for 5 minutes.

TO MAKE THE CHICKEN SALAD: Sprinkle chicken with salt and freshly ground black pepper to taste, then set aside.

If you are using canned chickpeas, drain and rinse them. In a small pan, sauté the chickpeas in olive oil over medium heat until slightly crisp.

In a large bowl, mix together the chicken, chickpeas, cabbage, dried fruit, and herbs. Top with the pickled onion and radish mixture and toss to combine.

Transfer to a large platter and finish with fresh-squeezed lemon juice, a drizzle of maple syrup, any remaining fresh herbs, and salt and pepper to taste.

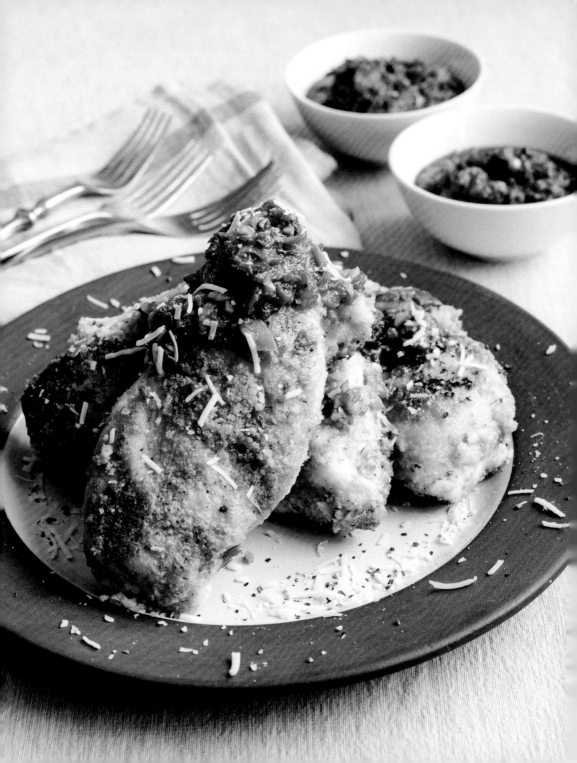

BAKED CHICKEN PARMESAN WITH BRIGHT & CHUNKY MARINARA

When you order chicken Parmesan at a restaurant, it tends to be soaked in olive oil and heavy on cheese. Here is a healthier version with a homemade marinara. Served with pasta, this dish could feed six people. If you really want to go all out, try the Fresh Spinach Pasta recipe that follows or the Homemade Egg Pasta recipe on p. xxx. To time it all just right, you'll want to start the pasta first. **Serves 4**

1 cup all-purpose flour
½ cup panko or other bread crumbs
1 tablespoon dried Italian herbs
    or seasoning mix
2 tablespoons freshly grated
    Parmesan, divided
4 medium-sized boneless, skinless
    chicken breasts
1 egg plus 1 tablespoon water,
    lightly beaten
2 tablespoons olive oil
1 cup shredded mozzarella
salt and pepper to taste

MARINARA

2 tablespoons olive oil
4 garlic cloves, minced
zest from half a lemon
2 cups diced red and green
    bell peppers
1 cup diced onion
1 large tomato, diced
¼ cup red wine vinegar
1 teaspoon brown sugar
½ cup chopped fresh parsley
1 28-ounce can crushed tomatoes
    or 4 cups tomatoes, chopped
salt and pepper to taste
juice from half a lemon
½ cup fresh basil leaves,
    cut into thick strips

Heat the oven to 375 degrees.

In a shallow bowl, mix together the flour, bread crumbs, Italian herbs or seasoning mix, and 1 tablespoon of the Parmesan. Lightly dust the chicken breasts with the flour and bread crumb mixture, brush with egg wash, and again dust with the flour mixture.

Heat the oil in a large ovenproof sauté pan over medium-high heat. Add chicken and cook for 4–5 minutes on each side until the breading is golden brown.

Transfer the pan to the oven to finish cooking while you make the marinara sauce. Cooking time will vary depending on the thickness of the chicken breasts—approximately 15–20 minutes, or until the juices run clear when you cut into the thickest part of the meat. You can also use a meat thermometer and cook until the meat reaches 165 degrees.

TO MAKE THE MARINARA: Warm the olive oil, garlic, and lemon zest in a large pot over medium-high heat. When the garlic begins to toast, stir in the peppers and onion and cook until they begin to soften, about 5 minutes. Then add the diced tomato and cook down for a couple of minutes.

(recipe continues)

Add in the red wine vinegar, brown sugar, and parsley and stir until completely combined. Add the crushed or chopped tomatoes and let cook another 5 minutes. Season to taste with salt, pepper, and lemon juice. Once you have removed the pot from the heat, fold in the fresh basil. Makes about 6 cups.

Transfer the chicken breasts to a large platter and sprinkle with salt, pepper, and mozzarella. Serve with individual bowls of marinara because the sauce is delicious on its own. Leftover marinara will keep for up to 3–4 days—it's great on top of most everything.

Note: To make this recipe gluten-free, use gluten-free panko crumbs and all-purpose gluten-free flour.

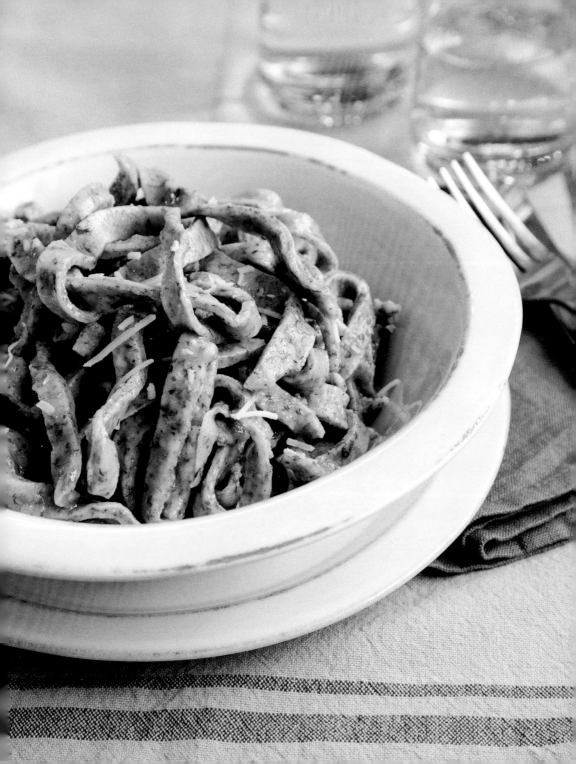

TECHNIQUE

FRESH SPINACH PASTA

There's something to be said for making fresh pasta in the simplest way, with your hands. But if it's your first time making spinach pasta, you might want to pull out the big guns if you have them tucked away in your pantry: A food processor and a pasta maker will make it much easier to incorporate the spinach and roll out the pasta. **Serves 8**

3 cups all-purpose flour
pinch of ground nutmeg
salt and pepper
8 ounces fresh spinach
2 eggs, plus 2 egg yolks
coarse semolina flour

This recipe yields approximately 2 pounds of cooked pasta. Fresh pasta is nearly twice as heavy as store-bought pasta, so the serving size will be about the same as 1 pound of dry pasta.

Add the flour, nutmeg, salt, and pepper into a large flat-bottomed bowl and make a well in the center.

Bring a large pot of salted water to a rolling boil over high heat. Immerse the spinach for up to 1 minute, and then immediately remove from heat while the color is still bright green. Reserve the water for cooking the fresh pasta, if desired.

Squeeze any excess water out of the spinach and then transfer it to a blender or food processor. Add the eggs and egg yolks and purée until you have a smooth paste.

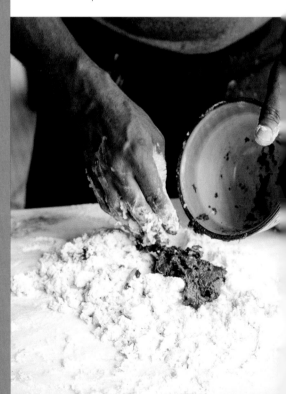

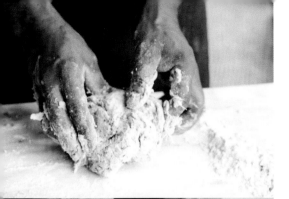

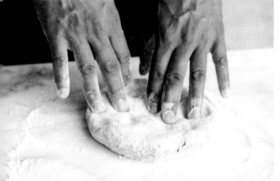

3

Roll out the pasta into thin, oblong sheets using a rolling pin or a pasta maker. Dust the work surface with semolina flour frequently to keep the dough from sticking.

To cut your pasta, roll up the flat sheet of dough tightly, starting from the shorter side. Use a sharp knife to cut into strips as wide as you would like. Cook on the stovetop in a large pot of salted water or reserved spinach water at a low rolling boil. Fresh pasta will float when it's fully cooked. Taste the noodles to make sure they are cooked to your liking. Fresh pasta will have a nice chewy texture.

2

Using a fork, mix the spinach and egg mixture into the flour little by little. The dough should be elastic and nonsticky. If it's not holding together, add in a splash of water. If it's still sticky, add a bit more flour. Once the mixture is thoroughly incorporated, cover and set it aside to rest for about 30 minutes at room temperature. This step allows the dough to relax so it will be easier to roll out and will give you a thinner pasta.

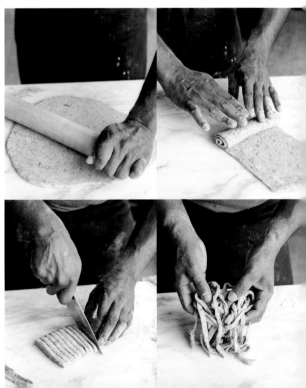

SPLIT CHICKEN WITH LEMON GARLIC SAUCE & ROASTED VEGETABLES

For this recipe you can purchase whole roasting chickens or any cuts that you like. When you go to the store, you will see different varieties of chicken—roaster, fryer, broiler. I say use whatever chicken you can catch. I typically plan for 4 ounces of cooked meat per person, so with 4 pounds of bone-in chicken, you might be lucky enough to have leftovers. Then fill the roasting pan with your favorite root vegetables. **Serves 6**

1 whole chicken, about
   4 pounds
olive oil
coarse salt and pepper
1 pound Brussels sprouts,
   cut in half
1 pound golden beets
   (about 3), peeled and
   sliced thick
½ bunch fresh parsley,
   coarsely chopped
4–6 garlic cloves
1 lemon, cut in half
2 teaspoons whole peppercorns

LEMON GARLIC SAUCE
pan-roasted lemons and garlic
2 tablespoons extra-virgin
   olive oil
juice from 1 lemon
salt and pepper to taste

Heat the oven to 375 degrees.

To split the chicken, set it on a cutting board, breast-side up. With a sharp, heavy knife, cut down the center. Flip it over and cut down either side of the backbone. Trim off any excess fat.

Brush lightly with olive oil and season with salt and pepper. Place the chicken, skin-side up, in a roasting pan. Let it come to room temperature as you prepare the vegetables.

Spread the cut vegetables, parsley, and garlic cloves around the roasting pan and lightly drizzle with additional olive oil, salt, and pepper. Place the lemon halves in the pan, cut-side up and add the peppercorns.

Bake for about 30 minutes on the middle rack of the oven. Remove to toss vegetables and brush the chicken with the liquid in the pan. Continue to bake for another 30 minutes or until the chicken is golden brown and the vegetables are tender. To get some additional color, increase the oven temperature to 400 degrees and move to the top rack of the oven to cook for the last 10 minutes. Remove from oven and allow the chicken to rest.

While the chicken is resting, remove roasted garlic cloves from pan and blend along with juice from the roasted lemons and extra-virgin olive oil. Add fresh lemon juice as needed and season to taste with salt and pepper. Drizzle over chicken and vegetables just before serving.

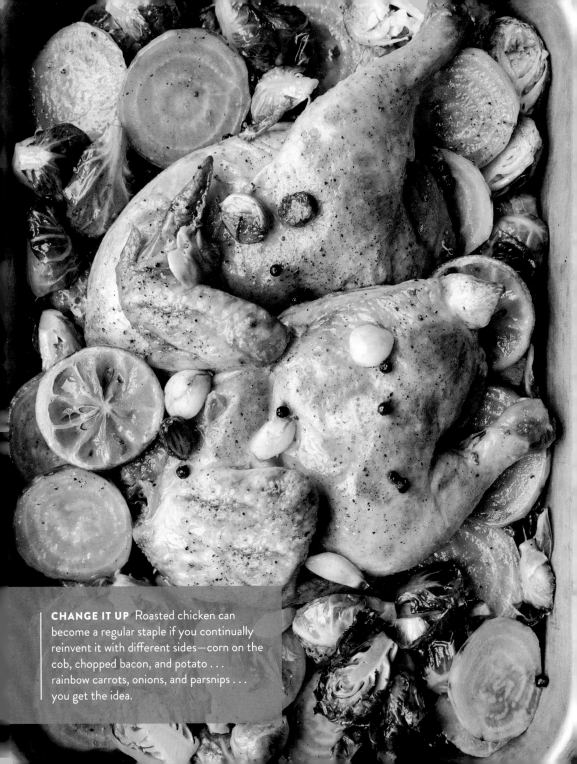

CHANGE IT UP Roasted chicken can become a regular staple if you continually reinvent it with different sides—corn on the cob, chopped bacon, and potato . . . rainbow carrots, onions, and parsnips . . . you get the idea.

CHICKEN PAD THAI

This is a light dish that balances fresh ingredients with a hint of heat and a subtle sweetness. Once you learn the timing of the different components, it's easy to make pad Thai at home in as little as 30 minutes. Best of all, you can dial in a flavor all your own. I like mine mild, without a lot of fish sauce. **Serves 4**

vegetable oil
2 pounds boneless, skinless
   chicken thighs, cut into
   bite-sized strips
salt and pepper to taste
8 ounces firm tofu,
   cut into cubes (optional)
2 eggs, lightly beaten
1 tablespoon sesame oil
8 ounces flat rice noodles
2 tablespoons chili paste or
   chili garlic sauce (Sambal,
   p. 196, also works well)
2 tablespoons low-sodium
   soy sauce
2 teaspoons fish sauce
8 ounces bean sprouts, divided
1 jalapeño, sliced
3 green onions, sliced thin

ON TOP
½ cup raw peanuts
2 tablespoons chopped fresh
   Thai basil and cilantro
crushed red pepper to taste
2 limes, cut into quarters
   lengthwise

Begin by toasting the peanuts for the topping in a dry pan over medium heat until they turn golden brown. Set aside to cool, then coarsely chop for topping.

Lightly coat the bottom of a large, shallow sauté pan with vegetable oil and cook the chicken thighs over medium heat with a sprinkle of salt and pepper. (If you are using tofu, add it here.) In a small bowl, lightly beat the eggs with the sesame oil. Once the chicken is nearly cooked through, add the egg mixture to the pan and scramble until dry. Set aside until you are ready to plate the noodles.

While the chicken is cooking, bring a large pot of water to a boil. Cook the rice noodles as directed on the package. Drain the noodles and toss them with a little sesame oil or water to prevent them from sticking.

Whisk together the chili paste or chili garlic sauce, soy sauce, and fish sauce in a large bowl. Add to the noodles along with half of the bean sprouts and the jalapeño and green onions and toss to coat.

Divide the noodle mixture between plates and top with the chicken and egg mixture. Finish with additional bean sprouts, fresh Thai basil and cilantro, toasted peanuts, crushed red pepper, and a couple of lime wedges.

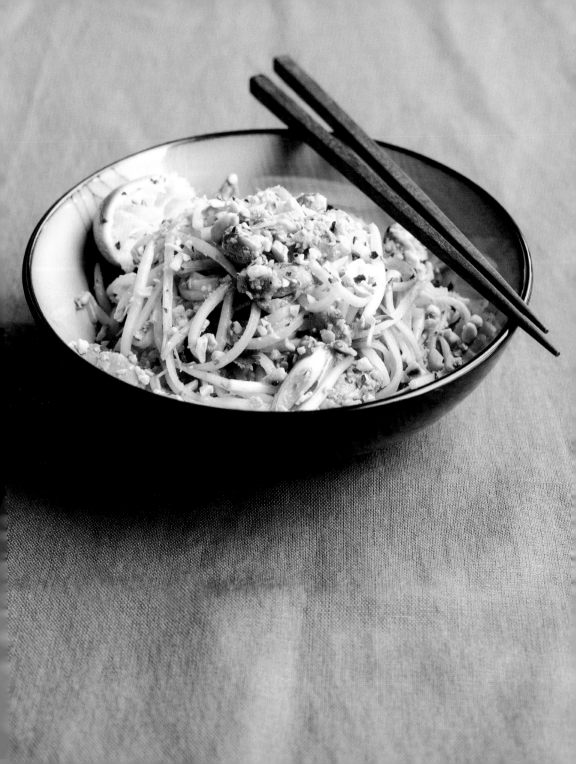

SAUTÉED TORTELLINI & SAUSAGE WITH COLLARD GREENS

When you sauté tortellini, it takes on a nice chewy texture, similar to a pot sticker. Finishing the pasta this way elevates a simple meal. If you "chiffonade" the collard greens, the finished dish is that much more impressive. Use a sharp knife to remove the rib, then roll up the leaves lengthwise and slice. **Serves 6**

1 pound fresh cheese tortellini
1 tablespoon olive oil
12 ounces chicken sausage
   links, cut into thin rounds
1 cup diced carrots
2 cups collard greens, ribs
   removed and thinly sliced
1 cup chicken stock
juice from half a lemon
2 tablespoons freshly
   grated Parmesan
drizzle of extra-virgin olive oil

Cook the tortellini in salted boiling water for about 5 minutes, or until they begin to float. Drain the pasta completely and spread out on a flat surface to cool.

In a sauté pan lightly coated in olive oil, toast the tortellini in small batches over medium heat. Once the edges are lightly browned, set aside.

Turn up the heat to medium-high and brown the sausage in the same pan. Add the carrots and cook for 1–2 minutes more.

Add the collard greens and stock. Bring to a low rolling boil, watching for the greens to brighten. Add the tortellini back into the pan and cook just long enough to heat.

Finish with a squeeze of lemon and serve with freshly grated Parmesan and a drizzle of olive oil.

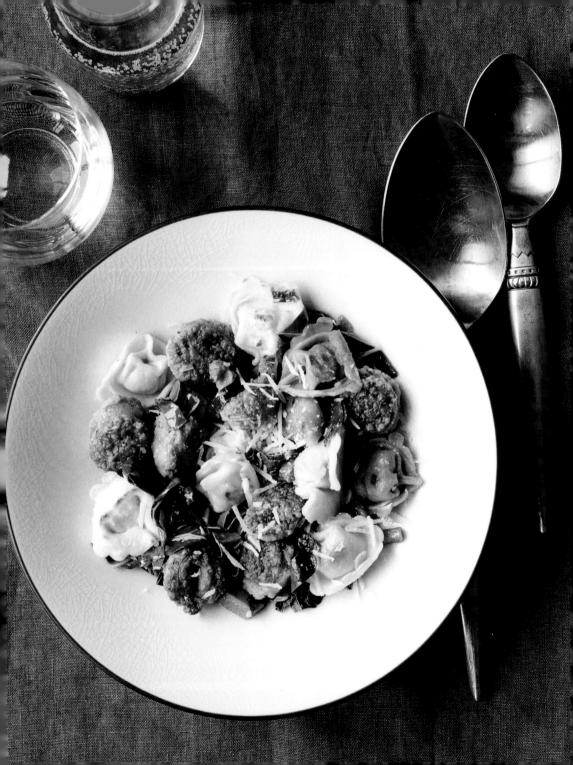

GRILLED CHICKEN WITH HOMEMADE BARBECUE SAUCE

This is one of my favorite fuss-free summertime recipes. Bone-in chicken is affordable and flavorful. Start with quality chicken leg quarters, the thigh and leg combo with the skin still on. Make the barbecue sauce ahead of time, and precook the chicken in the oven to make the prep even easier. **Serves 4**

4 chicken leg quarters
   (leg-thigh combo)
olive oil
salt and pepper to taste
½ cup Homemade Barbecue
   Sauce (p. 163), plus more
   for serving

Heat the oven to 400 degrees. Pat the chicken dry with paper towels, then rub with olive oil, salt, and pepper. Let rest for a few minutes to get to room temperature.

Bake the chicken for 30 minutes. Prepare the Homemade Barbecue Sauce (recipe follows) while the chicken is in the oven. Remove the chicken from the oven and store it in the fridge if you are grilling later.

Bring the grill to high heat. Grill the chicken skin-side down. Wait until you start to see the char marks, about 5 minutes, then flip. Once the chicken has been turned, brush it with barbecue sauce, and flip again after 4 more minutes. Continue to brush on barbecue sauce as needed.

After you have a good char going on each side, cut with a sharp knife to ensure the juices run clear or use a meat thermometer to check that the internal temperature has reached 165 degrees. Cover the chicken with foil and let rest a few minutes. Serve leg quarters whole or chop apart the drumstick and thigh before serving alongside a bowl of barbecue sauce.

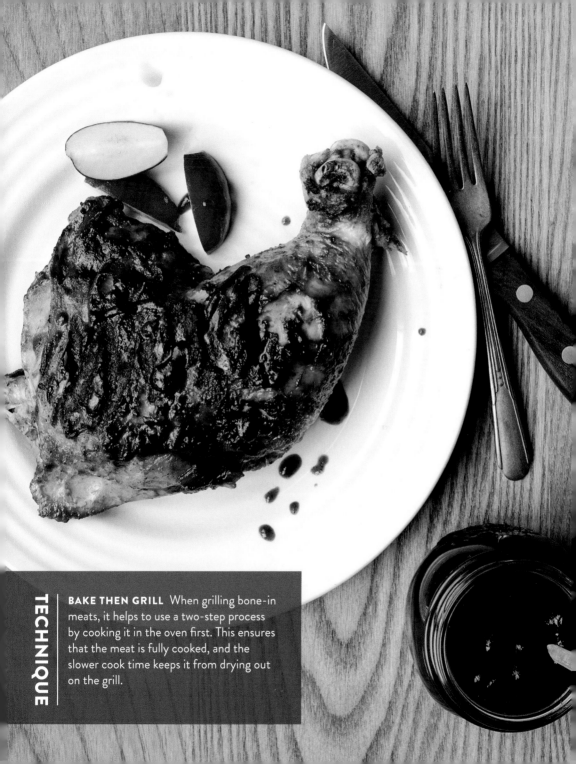

FRESH SAUCES

A fresh sauce adds flavor to anything you are making. Made with chopped herbs and vegetables, sauces can keep for up to one week if stored in the refrigerator. By replacing fresh ingredients such as ginger, garlic, and onion with dried herbs and spices, you can make a more shelf-stable sauce that will keep in the fridge much longer.

FRESH VS. DRIED

To swap out dried ingredients for fresh, use one-eighth of the measurement specified and adjust for flavor from there. The reverse goes for using fresh ingredients in place of dried herbs: You will need to use about eight times as much to get the same flavor.

WHERE TO LOOK

Dry herbs are not always found with the other spices. Look for dehydrated onions or garlic in the produce section. Some items, like dried cilantro and jalapeños, are shelved in specialty food sections.

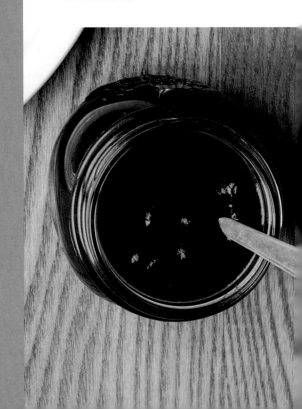

Homemade Barbecue Sauce

A good barbecue sauce is a balance of sweet and tangy heat. I like to use molasses, which gives this sauce its rich color and a more subtle sweetness. The tang comes from the red wine vinegar. The version that I've included here is more on the sweet side, which I've found to be a crowd-pleaser. **Makes 2 cups**

½ cup minced onion
   (or 1 tablespoon dried onions
   plus 2 tablespoons olive oil)
½ teaspoon garlic powder
1 teaspoon chili powder
½ teaspoon cinnamon
1 teaspoon coarsely ground
   black pepper
1 15-ounce can tomato sauce
¼ cup molasses
2 tablespoons brown sugar
¼ teaspoon salt
up to ½ cup red wine vinegar

Gently toast onions in a large pot over medium-high heat until they are dry. (If you are using dried onions, sauté in olive oil until golden brown.) Add the spices and stir while slowly adding tomato sauce—scrape the edges of the pan and keep a lid close by, as the splatter will be very hot.

Once the tomato sauce and spices have been thoroughly mixed together, add the molasses, brown sugar, and salt and continue to stir while drizzling in ¼ cup of the vinegar. Let simmer over medium heat for at least 15 minutes, or until the color darkens.

The flavor of tomato sauce and molasses can vary quite a bit. Adjust the flavor to your liking; if you want a more tangy flavor, add up to another ¼ cup of red wine vinegar. For a sweeter sauce, add more molasses or brown sugar, 1 tablespoon at a time.

Once you get it just right, remove from heat and let cool. As the sauce cools it will thicken and the flavors will continue to meld.

Store unused barbecue sauce in a sealed container in the fridge for up to 1 week.

CHANGE IT UP Next time, bring the heat. Grill a jalapeño and onion (cut in half, placed cut-side down on the grill) for about 5 minutes. Use in place of the dried or fresh onions.

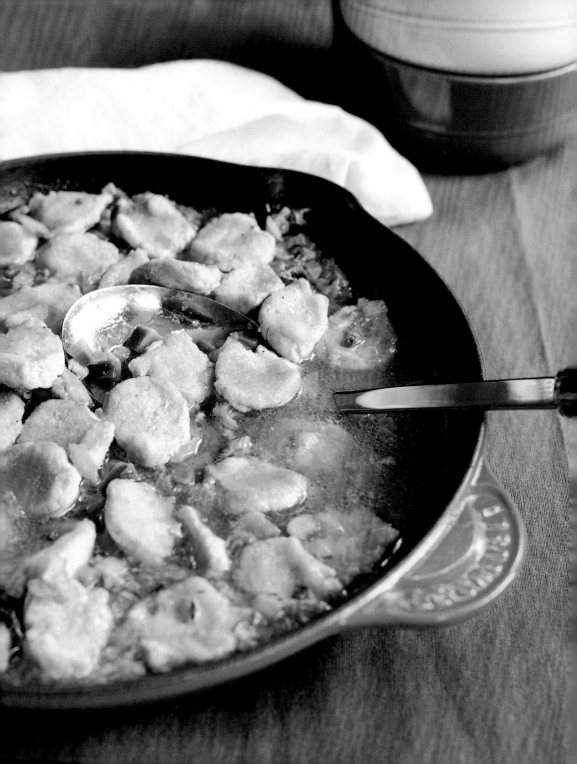

CHICKEN & ALMOND DUMPLINGS

This dish is yet another tribute to chicken pot pie—what's not to love? These dumplings use almond meal, which is really simple to work with, and it adds a comforting flavor and texture to this dish. It is also extra filling, thanks to the good fats and protein found in almonds. Serve up some homegrown love on a cool evening. **Serves 6**

1½ pounds boneless, skinless chicken thighs, cut into small pieces

¼ cup all-purpose gluten-free flour mixed with 1 teaspoon coarse salt and ½ teaspoon pepper

½ cup (3 ounces) coarsely chopped bacon

1 cup chopped onion

1 cup chopped carrots

1 cup chopped celery

1 quart chicken stock

1 teaspoon dry thyme

½ cup fresh herbs, such as thyme, parsley, and oregano (optional)

freshly grated Parmesan (optional)

ALMOND DUMPLINGS
2 cups almond meal

2 eggs, lightly beaten

½ teaspoon ground nutmeg

dash of cinnamon

Heat the oven to 350 degrees.

In a large bowl, combine the almond dumpling ingredients. Stir until the mixture comes together as a thick dough. If it's too dry, drizzle in warm water as needed, 1 teaspoon at a time. Set aside to rest while you cook the chicken.

Lightly dust the chicken in the flour mixture. Heat a deep oven-safe sauté pan over medium-high heat and add the bacon. Cook for a couple of minutes to give the bacon a head start. Add the chicken, and cook for 5–6 minutes, stirring occasionally, until it's lightly browned. Next, stir in the onions, carrots, and celery and cook until they begin to soften. By now the bacon should be crispy. Add the stock and thyme and bring to a slow rolling boil.

Pinch off small pieces of the dumpling dough and drop into the hot broth. Finish the dish in the oven, baking for 20 minutes, or until the dumplings begin to absorb the liquid and puff up slightly. Ladle into bowls and top with fresh herbs and Parmesan cheese, if desired.

CHICKEN MADRAS & YOGURT SAUCE WITH HARISSA

This dish borrows from a few cultures to give us one of our favorite flavor combinations— a little spice, some roasted warmth, and cool yogurt. For an extra kick of flavor, serve with Harissa, see p. 168. **Serves 6**

4 pounds bone-in, skin-on
  chicken thighs
1 cup thinly sliced onion
2 jalapeños, sliced into
  thin strips
1 large tomato, cut in half
  and sliced thin
8 ounces mushrooms,
  cut in half
2 tablespoons Madras
  curry powder
2 tablespoons coconut oil,
  melted
1 teaspoon coarse salt
½ teaspoon coarsely
  ground black pepper
1 lemon, cut in half

YOGURT SAUCE
1 cup plain yogurt
1 tablespoon minced jalapeño
1 tablespoon minced shallots
  or red onion
1 tablespoon chopped
  fresh cilantro
salt to taste
juice from half a lemon
extra-virgin olive oil

Heat the oven to 400 degrees.

Trim off any excess fat or skin from the chicken and set the chicken aside. Mix the vegetables, curry powder, coconut oil, and salt and pepper in a large bowl. Add the chicken and rub it thoroughly with the spice mix.

Transfer everything into an oven-safe baking dish, making sure the chicken is skin-side down. Bake for 30 minutes.

Scrape the pan, mixing the vegetables, flip the chicken over, and bake skin-side up on the top rack of the oven for another 15 minutes, or until the skin crisps and juices run clear.

TO MAKE THE YOGURT SAUCE: While the chicken is baking, place yogurt, jalapeño, shallots or onion, and cilantro in a blender and pulse until smooth. Adjust for flavor with salt, lemon juice, and olive oil, as needed. Chill until you are ready to serve. (Leftover yogurt sauce can be kept in the fridge for 2–3 days.)

Just before serving, top the chicken with a squeeze of fresh lemon and a dollop of yogurt sauce.

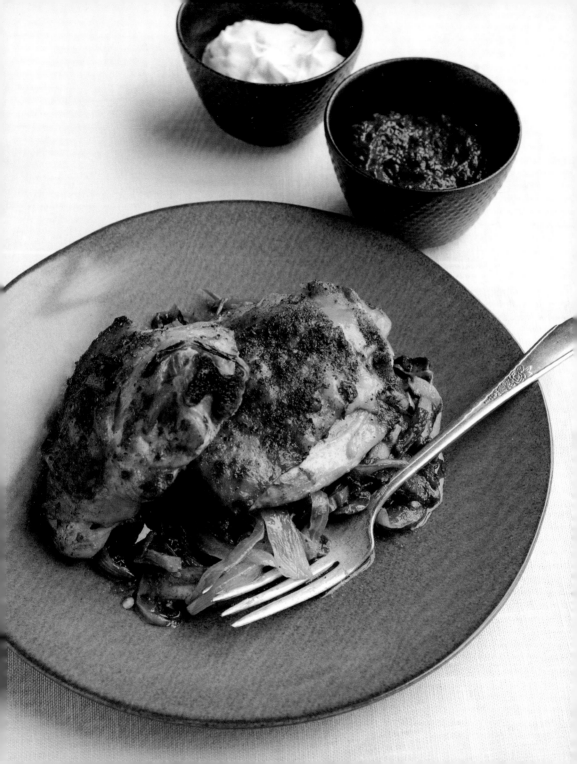

Harissa

This is a classic North African sauce made from ground spices, to be used in the same way as moles, pestos, and chutneys from all over the world. Use the ingredients you have available and add in the chiles you can handle, then load up on garlic, lemon juice, and olive oil. • Look for dried cilantro in the Mexican section of your local grocery store. Dried mint is often there as well, or is readily available at Middle Eastern markets. **Makes 1½–2 cups**

5 dry ancho chiles
5 dry guajillo chiles
1 tablespoon whole
   coriander seeds
1 tablespoon paprika
1 teaspoon cumin seeds
1 teaspoon dry mint leaves
1 teaspoon dry cilantro
4–5 garlic cloves
¼ cup extra-virgin olive oil
1 tablespoon apple
   cider vinegar
1 teaspoon coarse salt
juice from 2 lemons

Bring a small pot or tea kettle of water to boil. Place the chiles in a bowl and pour the boiling water over them until submerged. Cover with a lid or plastic wrap and let rest for 10–15 minutes, until the skin peels off easily. Drain, peel, remove any seeds and stems, and set aside.

Gently toast the spices and herbs in a dry pan over medium-high heat until they become very fragrant— about 5 minutes should be enough. Stir consistently to keep from scorching. Remove from heat.

Combine the garlic cloves, olive oil, vinegar, and salt in a blender along with your dry toasted spice mix and chiles. Pulse as you drizzle in the lemon juice until the mixture becomes a smooth paste. Adjust flavor with lemon and salt to taste.

Store in an airtight container in the fridge for up to 2 weeks.

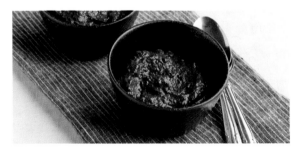

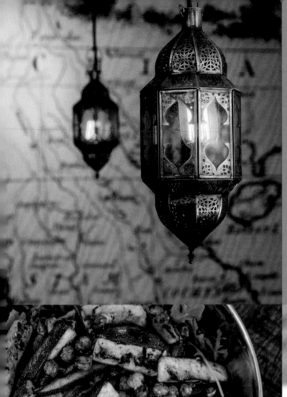

Small details can shape our experience of a meal. Look to simple, inexpensive things you can do to make a meal seem special. Food doesn't have to be fussy to taste great.

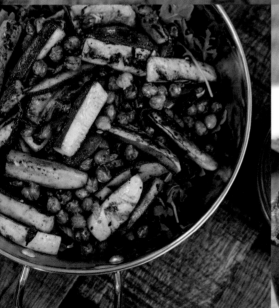

MAKE AN IMPRESSION

RED CHICKEN
WITH BAKED BIRIYANI

This fragrant and colorful dish can easily feed a large group. Beets were traditionally used in dishes like tandoori chicken to get that vibrant red color. I think you'll find this made-from-scratch marinade is well worth your time. **Serves 8**

8 chicken drumsticks
1 cup plain whole-milk yogurt
1 small red beet,
    peeled and diced
1 teaspoon minced fresh ginger
1 teaspoon minced garlic
½ teaspoon cayenne
1 tablespoon Madras
    curry powder
1 tablespoon sweet paprika
1½ teaspoons coarse salt
juice from 1 lemon
salt and pepper to taste

BAKED BIRIYANI

3 cups uncooked basmati rice
2 cups water
1 cup frozen mixed peas
    and carrots
½ cup raisins
2 tablespoons chopped
    cashews or peanuts
2 jalapeños, sliced into thin
    strips (remove seeds for
    a milder flavor)
4 bay leaves
1 teaspoon ground cinnamon
1 tablespoon Madras curry
    powder
1 teaspoon coarse salt

Prep the chicken by trimming off the excess fat. Remove the nubby ends of the drumsticks with a sharp knife—with a firm whack the ends will pop right off, making it easy to remove the skin and giving the dish a more finished look. Place the drumsticks in a baking dish and set aside.

In a blender or food processor combine the yogurt, beet, ginger, garlic, spices, salt, and purée. The yogurt mixture will be a bright red color.

Thoroughly coat the chicken with the yogurt mixture. Chill for at least 30 minutes or overnight to let the meat soak up the flavor.

Heat the oven to 350 degrees.

To make the biriyani, rinse the rice in a strainer until the water runs clear. Place the rice directly into a large baking dish (approximately 9 × 13–inch). Add the remaining biriyani ingredients and gently stir until the spices are evenly distributed. Cover with foil and place on the middle rack of the oven. Starting the chicken separately in the oven maintains their distinct colors and flavors.

After the rice has cooked for 15 minutes, cover the chicken with foil and bake for approximately 45 minutes.

Remove the chicken and the biriyani from the oven. Pour off the excess marinade from the chicken and reserve for serving, if desired. Fluff the biriyani with a wooden spoon and lay the drumsticks on top. Return to the oven to bake uncovered for another 20 minutes, or until rice is fully cooked. Finish with lemon juice and sprinkle with salt and pepper to taste.

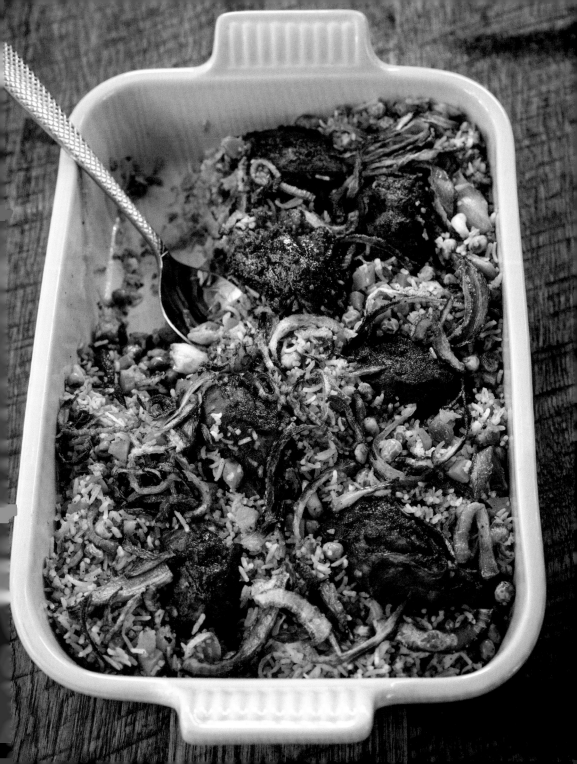

Roasted Tomato Yogurt Sauce

You can achieve that warm-roasted tomato taste by using a hot grill, frying pan, or the oven broiler. Change up the peppers to get the heat that is right for you. **Makes 3 cups**

2 medium tomatoes
1 jalapeño or your favorite
   pepper
2 cloves garlic
1 tablespoon coconut oil,
   melted
salt to taste
2 cups plain yogurt
small handful of cilantro
juice from half a lemon

Remove the stems from the tomatoes and jalapeño and cut lengthwise. You can remove the seeds from the pepper to keep the flavor milder.

Brush the tomatoes, jalapeño, and garlic with oil and sprinkle with salt. Grill, broil, or toss into a very hot frying pan until the skin blisters and begins to get a nice char in places; just a few minutes is all it takes. Remove from heat and let cool.

Transfer the roasted vegetables into a blender and add yogurt, along with a pinch of salt and cilantro.

Before serving, add a squeeze of fresh lemon and further season with salt to taste.

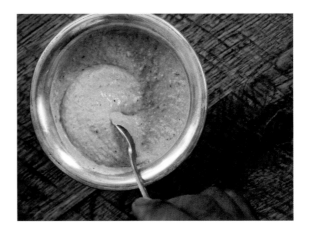

PAIRS WELL WITH FALAFEL (P. 262) AND WARM PITAS.

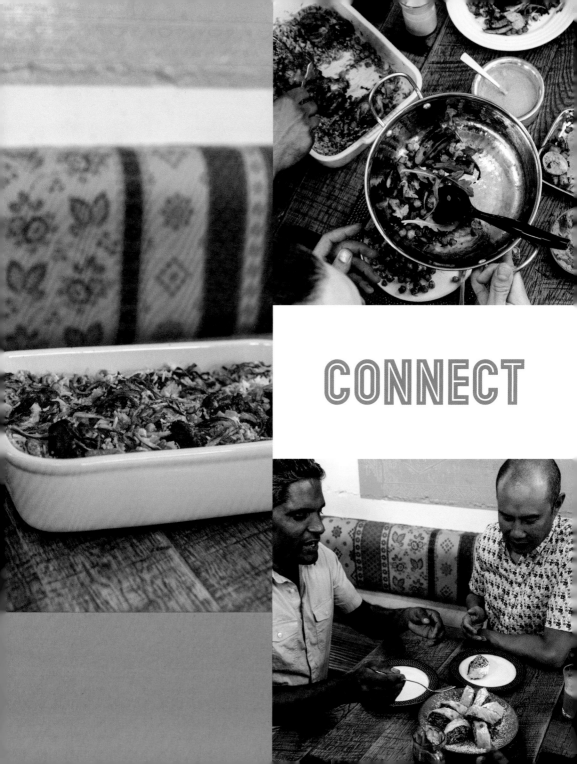

CONNECT

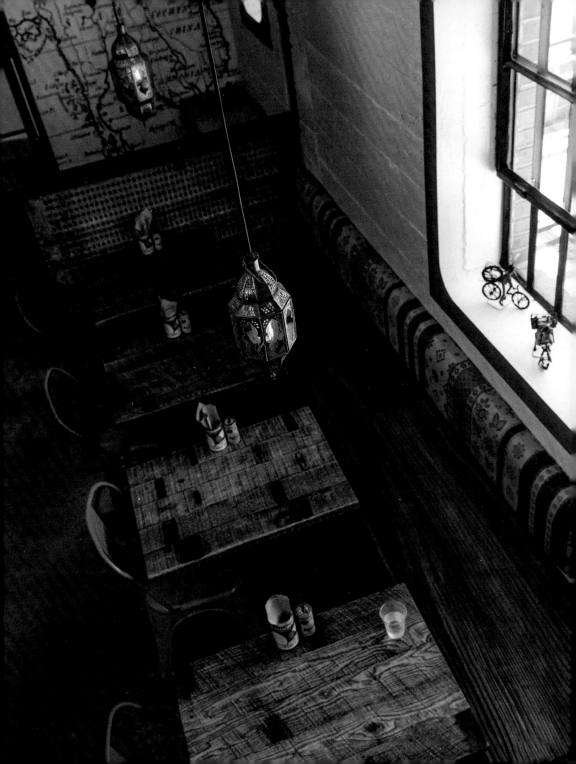

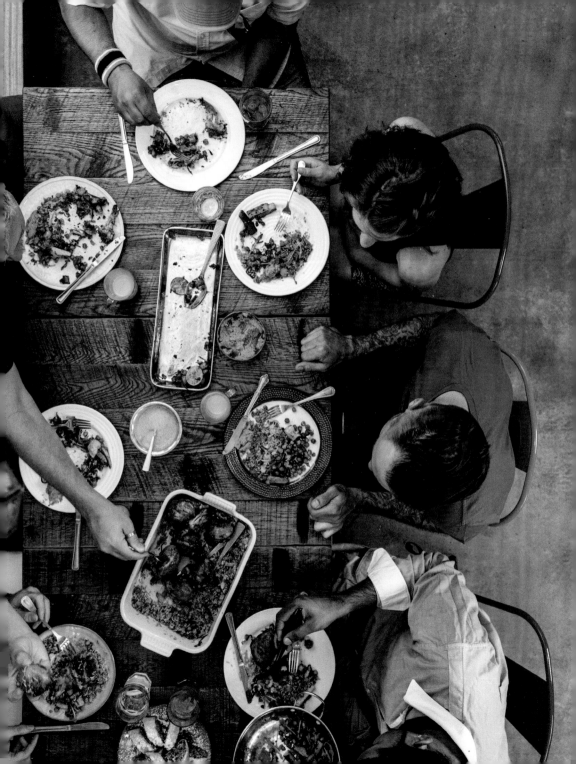

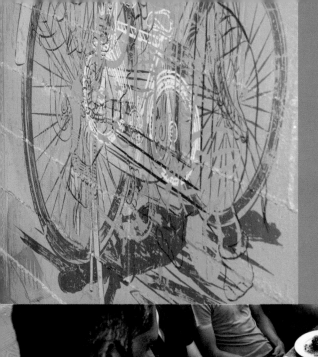

We inherit culture from our families and then choose what to carry forward. Flavors rooted in personal experience are powerful. Biju's curry is a compelling taste of home, regardless of where you come from.

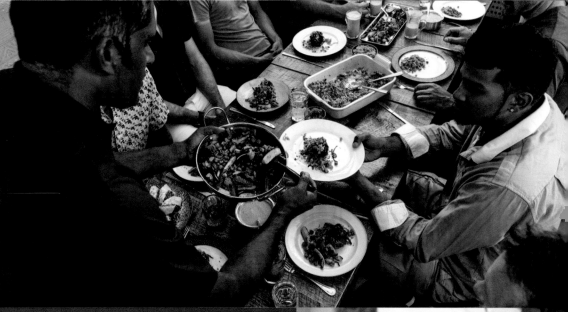

PASS IT FORWARD

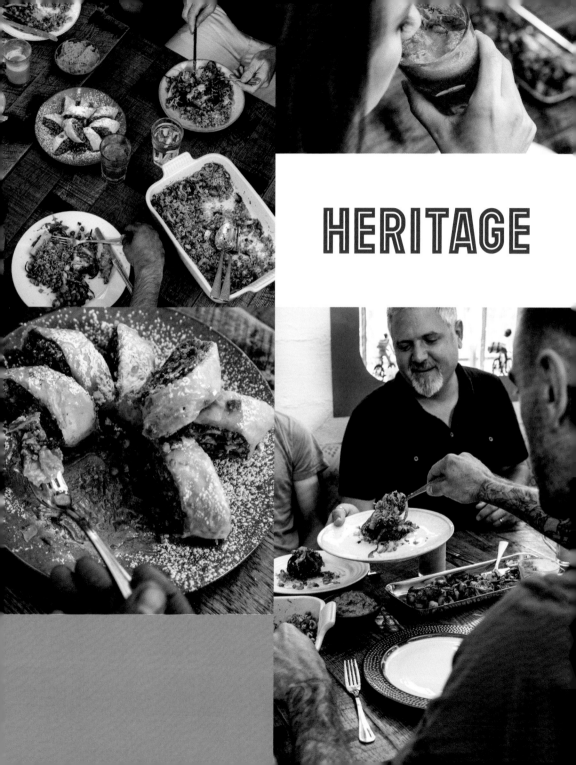

HERITAGE

SEA CHANGE

*Unless you've grown up with it, seafood can
be intimidating. Here are a few basics
to build into your repertoire so you can say goodbye
to canned tuna and fish sticks once and for all.*

SEAFOOD

BAKED JAMBALAYA

Jambalaya involves a lot of steps—and the steps matter—but you will master this dish quickly. All you need is a dark roux, salty meat, some vegetables, rice, and shellfish. While it traditionally uses shrimp and mussels, you can use whatever seafood you have access to. If fresh seafood is hard to come by, smoked oysters work well. **Serves 6**

2 cups (about 12 ounces) smoked sausage or bacon, cut into bite-sized chunks
½ cup chopped onion
½ pound medium-sized shrimp (about 10–16), peeled and deveined, or a 3-ounce tin smoked oysters, drained
1 cup chopped celery
1 cup chopped red bell pepper
1 cup diced carrots
1 cup crushed tomatoes
3 cloves minced garlic
4 sprigs fresh thyme, stems removed
¼ cup coarsely chopped fresh parsley
2 cups uncooked short-grain rice (jasmine or any nonsticky rice)
4 cups water or chicken stock
3–4 bay leaves
½ pound mussels, cleaned
up to 1 teaspoon salt
drizzle of extra-virgin olive oil
freshly grated Parmesan

ROUX
½ cup (1 stick) butter
1 cup all-purpose flour

Heat the oven to 350 degrees.

While the oven is heating, start your roux in a large cast-iron or oven-safe sauté pan. Melt the butter over medium heat. Stir in the flour with a wooden spoon and turn up the heat to medium-high. Continue stirring and scraping the mixture together as it cooks until the color darkens into a nice golden brown.

Scrape the roux into a bowl and set aside. In the same pan, brown the sausage or bacon, then add the onions and cook until they are translucent and slightly browned.

Reduce the heat to medium, add the shrimp, and sauté until they turn pink, just a few minutes. If you are using smoked oysters instead, add them now.

Incorporate half of the roux into the mixture. Now add in the celery, red bell pepper, carrots, tomatoes, garlic, and fresh herbs and cook for about 5 minutes.

Stir in the rice and water or stock, along with bay leaves. Fold in the mussels, cover the pot, and transfer to the oven. Bake for 30 minutes, then check to see if the rice is cooked. Add more water in ¼ cup increments if needed and bake until cooked off.

Season to taste with salt, if needed, and finish with olive oil and freshly grated Parmesan.

Note: If you want more sauce next time around, increase the roux and add equal parts of water or stock. For every tablespoon of roux added, use 1 cup of water or stock.

COOKING WITH MUSSELS To clean mussels, scrub the outer shell to remove any fuzzy bits and dirt. Open mussels should be discarded. If you have some mussels that don't open after cooking, those will need to be discarded as well.

HOW TO USE ROUX This recipe uses just half of the roux prepared. Tightly wrap the remaining roux in plastic wrap and store in the fridge to use as a base or thickener for other cooked sauces. The roux will keep in the fridge for up to 4 weeks.

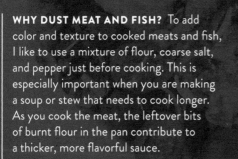

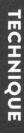

TECHNIQUE

WHY DUST MEAT AND FISH? To add color and texture to cooked meats and fish, I like to use a mixture of flour, coarse salt, and pepper just before cooking. This is especially important when you are making a soup or stew that needs to cook longer. As you cook the meat, the leftover bits of burnt flour in the pan contribute to a thicker, more flavorful sauce.

For dusting, I recommend all-purpose gluten-free flour because it has a slightly more nutty, rich flavor while yielding the same results as regular all-purpose flour. While most of our recipes don't specify gluten-free flour, it can be used in most every recipe calling for all-purpose flour.

CATFISH PICCATA

What we love about piccata is the bright and briny flavors of the white wine and capers. Here is a simple, fast version that you can serve over pasta or by itself for a delicious low-carb alternative. **Serves 4**

1 pound skinless catfish filets
¼ cup all-purpose flour mixed
    with 1 teaspoon Italian
    seasoning, 1 teaspoon coarse
    salt, and ½ teaspoon pepper
2 tablespoons olive oil
½ cup shallot or red onion,
    thinly sliced
2 cloves garlic, minced
1 cup dry white wine
1 pint cherry tomatoes
2 tablespoons capers, drained
¼ cup coarsely chopped basil
juice from 1 lemon, divided
2 tablespoons butter
coarse salt and pepper to taste

ON TOP
1 tablespoon chopped
    fresh parsley
1 teaspoon chopped fresh
    thyme (optional)

Rinse and pat dry the catfish filets with paper towels, then dust them in the mixture of flour, Italian seasoning, salt, and pepper. Shake gently to remove extra flour.

Heat the olive oil in a large sauté pan over high heat, then add the catfish filets and sear until golden brown, about 3 minutes on each side. Remove the fish from the pan.

Add the shallot or red onion and garlic and quickly brown. Then add the white wine, tomatoes, capers, basil, half the lemon juice, and bring to a low boil.

Finish by incorporating the remaining lemon juice and butter into the hot pan for added richness. Adjust flavor with salt and pepper. Top with fresh herbs.

GRILLED SALMON STEAK SANDWICHES

Next time you plan a game-day party or summertime lunch, serve up a platter of these sandwiches. Salmon steaks are a beautiful substitute for burgers—they are every bit as accessible on a bun. The Mustard Yogurt Dressing and fresh green salad make each bite even more delicious. **Serves 4**

4 pieces of salmon
   (about 1 pound)
1 tablespoon olive oil
salt and pepper to taste
4 ciabatta rolls or 1 large
   crusty baguette
2 cups bitter greens such
   as arugula
half an English cucumber,
   cut in half lengthwise and
   thinly sliced
¼ cup thinly sliced red onion
juice from half a lemon
½ teaspoon coarse salt

MUSTARD YOGURT DRESSING

½ cup thick plain Greek yogurt
2 tablespoons coarse-ground
   mustard
1 teaspoon extra-virgin olive oil
1 tablespoon capers, drained
juice from half a lemon
1 teaspoon red pepper flakes
salt and pepper to taste

Heat the grill (or see note below). While the grill is getting nice and hot, brush the salmon with olive oil and season generously with salt and pepper. Place salmon skin-side down on grill. Cook for about 5 minutes, then gently flip and cook for another 4–5 minutes. The salmon should have a nice char on the outside and be cooked to medium, an internal temperature of 145 degrees.

While the salmon is cooking, slice the ciabatta rolls or baguette and warm on the grill.

Combine greens, cucumber, and onion in a bowl. Dress with the lemon juice, coarse salt, and pepper to taste.

TO MAKE THE DRESSING: In a small bowl whisk together the ingredients for the mustard dressing until smooth.

Generously spread the dressing on the bread and assemble the sandwiches with the salmon steaks and arugula mixture. Serve immediately.

Note: You can also cook the salmon on the stovetop in a heavy sauté pan over medium-high heat.

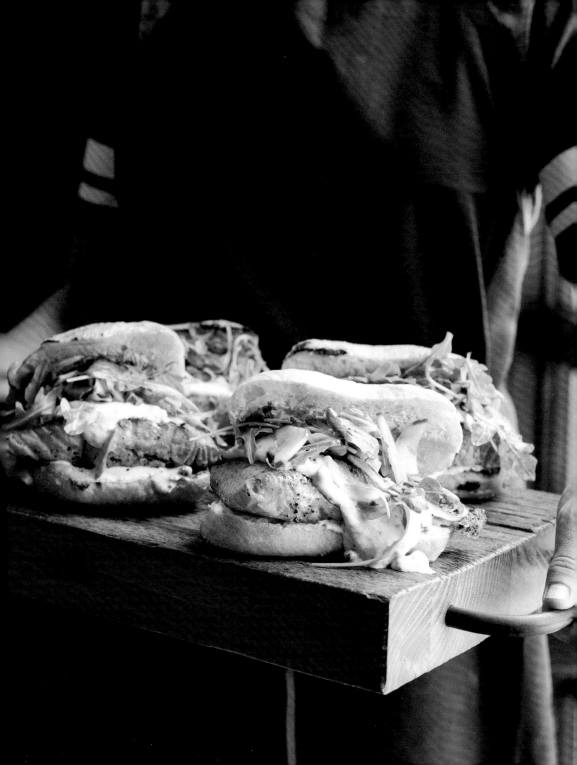

MISO & MAPLE-MARINATED COD WITH SWEET PEA RISOTTO

This is a simplified version of the classic miso-marinated black cod made famous in the United States by Master Sushi Chef Nobu Matsuhisa. The cod works best when cooked under the broiler with the heat blasting down. You can also prepare it in a pan on the stovetop or on a grill. Cod is a delicate fish—in fact, as it cooks you will see the layers begin to separate a bit. For this reason, avoid flipping during the cooking time. Keep in mind the side you want to present, and make sure to cook that side up. This creamy risotto pairs beautifully with the fish. **Serves 6**

6 thick pieces of cod or
   any other white fish
   (about 3 pounds)
½ cup maple syrup
2 tablespoons white
   miso paste
1 tablespoon grated
   fresh ginger
1 teaspoon sesame oil
coarse salt and pepper to taste
2 teaspoons lemon zest
juice from 1 lemon

SWEET PEA RISOTTO

6 cups chicken stock
2 tablespoons olive oil or
   butter, plus additional
   to taste
2 cups arborio or risotto rice
2 cloves garlic, minced
1 cup dry white wine
2 cups fresh or frozen peas
¼ cup freshly grated Parmesan
zest from half a lemon
coarse salt and pepper to taste

Place the fish in an oven-safe baking dish with some space between each piece. Mix all the remaining ingredients together in a small bowl. Brush the fish generously with the marinade, cover, and refrigerate while you prepare the risotto. (If you have the time, you can let it marinate overnight.)

TO MAKE THE RISOTTO: In a saucepan, bring the stock to a boil, then reduce heat and let simmer. This will speed up the cook time. Warm the olive oil or butter in a heavy pot over medium heat. Add the rice and garlic and gently toast, taking care not to let it smoke or burn. The rice will become translucent as it soaks up the oil or butter. As it begins to brown, add the white wine, stirring continually until the liquid has evaporated. Reduce heat to medium-low and add 2 cups of warm stock, stirring periodically until fully absorbed, about 10–15 minutes. Then add another 2 cups of stock and let the mixture cook down again, approximately another 10 minutes. The risotto will thicken as the stock is absorbed. Add the remaining stock and stir until you have a creamy risotto. The risotto will continue to absorb liquid as it sits, so use a bit more stock than you think you need.

(recipe continues)

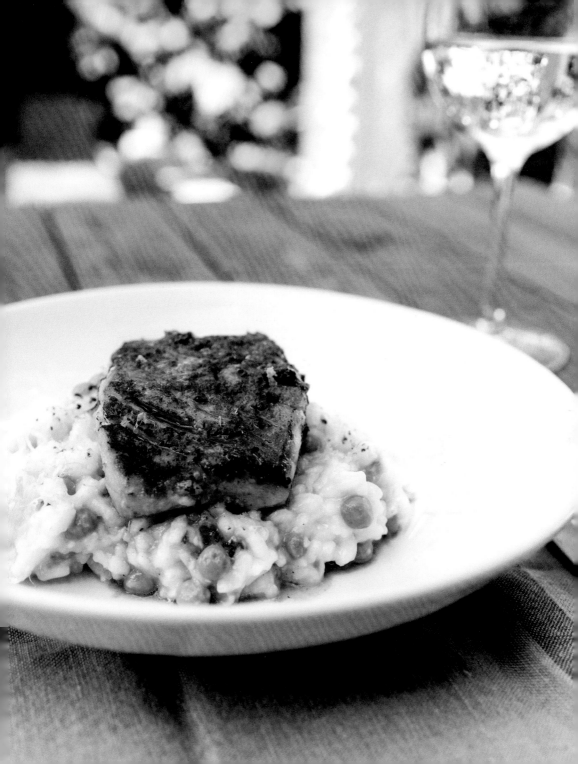

Add in the peas, Parmesan, and lemon zest. Season to taste with salt and pepper and additional olive oil or butter, if desired. Remove from heat and keep covered until ready to serve.

TO COOK THE COD: Heat the broiler to high. Place the cod under the broiler for about 8–10 minutes, or until the marinade takes on a light char and the cod begins to flake. Let the fish rest for about a minute and serve with risotto while still warm.

CHANGE IT UP You can also use 1 cup leftover salty meats like prosciutto to make a more savory risotto. Pair with a hearty vegetable such as asparagus or broccoli florets. Add blanched vegetables and meat in place of peas and lemon zest.

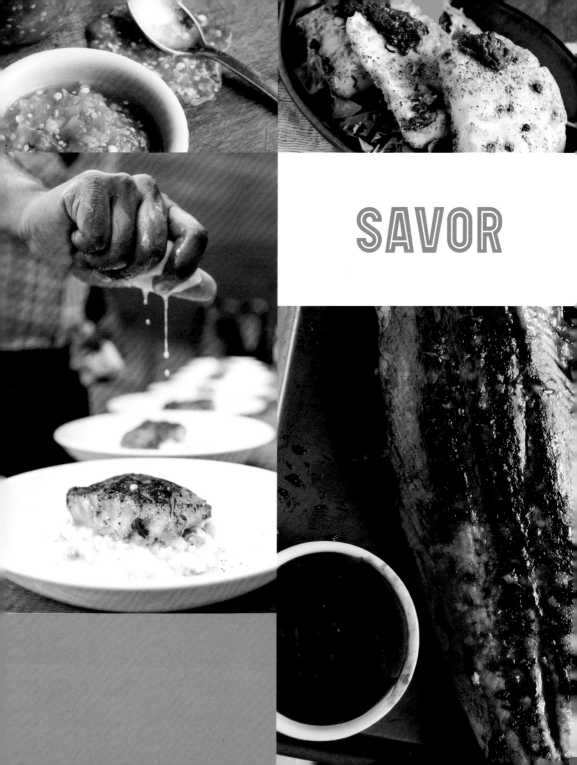

SAVOR

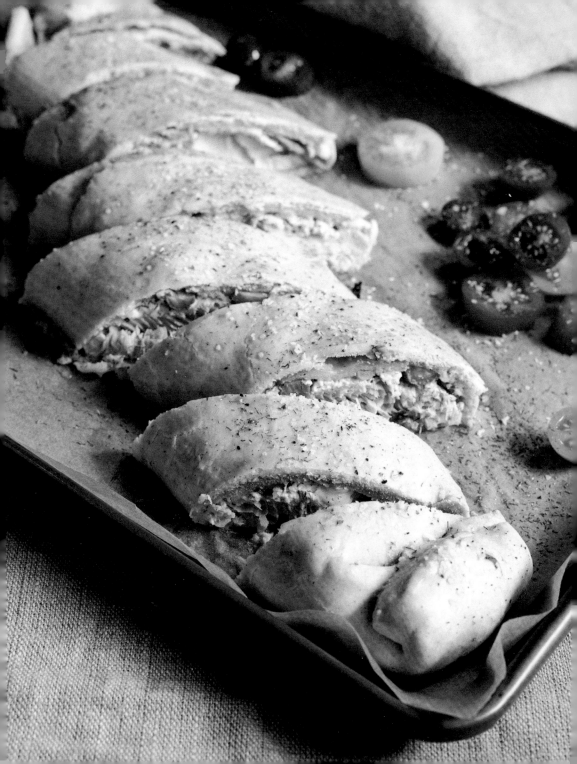

BAKED SALMON
IN PASTRY

This is an elegant main dish that you can pull out for the holidays or any special occasion. Preserves, pickles, and yogurt are familiar ingredients that you likely already have on hand. A golden-brown pastry is the key to getting it right. If you don't have time to make the pastry from scratch, look for a high-quality store-bought puff pastry or piecrust. **Serves 8**

1 large boneless, skinless
    salmon filet, about 2 pounds
coarse salt and pepper to taste
2 tablespoons peach or
    apricot preserves
½ cup plain Greek yogurt
¼ cup thinly sliced cornichons
    (sliced lengthwise)
1 teaspoon dry dill
1 egg plus a splash of water,
    lightly beaten

PASTRY
1½ cups all-purpose flour
¼ teaspoon salt
¼ teaspoon ground cinnamon
⅓ cup cold butter, cut into
    ½-inch cubes
½ cup cold water

ON TOP
1 cup sliced cherry tomatoes
1 lemon, sliced

TO MAKE THE PASTRY: In a food processor or standing mixer, combine the flour, salt, and cinnamon. Add butter and blend until the butter is incorporated into a crumbly mixture.

With the food processor or mixer running, add cold water a little bit at a time. Use a spatula to periodically scrape down the sides of the bowl until the flour is completely worked into the dough. Press dough together into an oblong disk and wrap tightly in plastic wrap. Chill in the fridge for at least 30 minutes before rolling out the pastry.

TO PREPARE THE FISH: While the pastry is chilling, take the salmon out of the fridge. Remove the skin and bones, if any. Season the salmon lightly with coarse salt and pepper and let warm to room temperature.

Heat the oven to 350 degrees.

To assemble, remove the pastry from the fridge. Keep in mind that cold butter can be a little hard to work with—take your time rolling the dough out, and it will warm up. Place a sheet of parchment paper on your work surface and sprinkle it lightly with flour. Roll the dough into a rectangle long enough to wrap the salmon. Use the parchment paper to lift the pastry onto a baking sheet. Place the salmon filet on the center of the pastry.

(recipe continues)

Brush the preserves onto the salmon, followed by the yogurt. Top with cornichons, and then sprinkle with dill. Fold the pastry dough over the top of the filet and brush the pastry with a little egg wash where it will seal. Pinch the edges of the pastry together, then gently position it so the seam is underneath the filet. Trim off any excess dough with a sharp knife.

Brush the top of the pastry with egg wash and cut a few slits into the top of the dough to allow the steam to vent during baking. The egg wash will help you know when the crust is cooked.

Baking time will vary depending on the size of the salmon. When the pastry has a nice golden brown color—at approximately 30–35 minutes—remove it from the oven and let it rest. Use a meat thermometer to be absolutely sure it's done. Cook until the internal temperature of the salmon reaches 145 degrees.

Serve with sliced tomatoes and lemon or any other garden-fresh vegetables you have on hand.

DELICIOUS WITH OLIVE OIL-POACHED TOMATO SOUP (P. 110) IN WINTER OR FRESH GRAPEFRUIT AND AVOCADO SALAD (P. 113) IN SPRING AND SUMMER.

LOBSTER MAC 'N' CHEESE WITH FRESH TOMATILLO SAUCE

Consider this a pot of recovery—it's an indulgent take on mac 'n' cheese for grown-ups. Frozen or canned lobster will work just fine in a dish like this one. I typically find higher-quality frozen lobster meat at the fish counter. With a cheesy sauce like this, I like to use a shorter noodle, whether penne or a curly or twisty variety. **Serves 4**

8 ounces cooked lobster
8 ounces uncooked pasta (rotini, penne, or your favorite shape)
2 tablespoons butter
1 cup minced celery
¼ cup minced onion
2 cloves garlic, minced
½ cup all-purpose flour or rice flour
2 cups milk
1 cup shredded Vermont sharp white cheddar
1 cup shredded Gruyère
dash of nutmeg
¼ teaspoon celery salt
coarse salt and pepper to taste
2 tablespoons chopped fresh herbs (chives, parsley, thyme, dill)
juice from 1 lemon

If the lobster is frozen, let it thaw in the refrigerator, then tip out any excess liquid.

Bring a large pot of salted water to a boil and prepare the pasta as directed on the package. Drain the pasta and set it aside.

Melt the butter in a sauté pan over medium-high heat, then add the celery, onions, and garlic. Cook until the onions soften and turn golden brown, about 4–5 minutes. Add the flour to make a roux, scraping the bottom of the pan with a spatula.

Reduce the heat to medium and add the milk, whisking to get a consistent mixture. Keep stirring until it begins to thicken.

Reduce the heat to low and stir in the cheddar and Gruyère, nutmeg, and celery salt until the cheese melts and the seasoning is fully incorporated. Taste and season further with salt and pepper as needed. Gently fold in lobster and pasta, cooking just long enough to heat.

Serve in individual bowls and finish with fresh herbs and lemon juice.

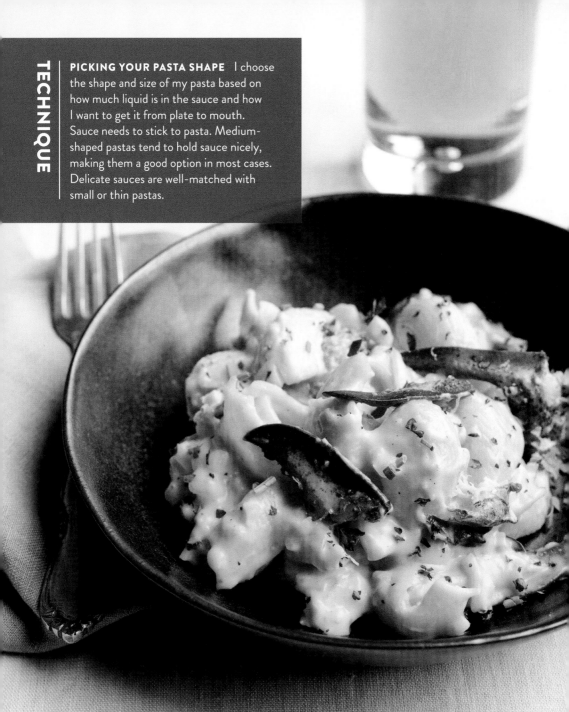

PICKING YOUR PASTA SHAPE I choose the shape and size of my pasta based on how much liquid is in the sauce and how I want to get it from plate to mouth. Sauce needs to stick to pasta. Medium-shaped pastas tend to hold sauce nicely, making them a good option in most cases. Delicate sauces are well-matched with small or thin pastas.

Fresh Tomatillo Sauce

Tomatillos have a somewhat tart taste and just enough acidity to balance out a rich meal. If you can't resist a little heat, take 10 minutes to make this fresh sauce. **Makes 4 cups**

1 pound tomatillos
2 jalapeños, destemmed
1 teaspoon salt

Bring a pot of water to a rolling boil and drop in the tomatillos. Cook for 5 minutes to blanch the fruit. Drain the water and remove the husks. Transfer the tomatillos to a food processor or blender. Add in the jalapeños and salt. (To create a more mild flavor, remove the seeds from the peppers.) Coarsely chop for a chunky texture.

Store leftover sauce in the fridge in an airtight container for up to 1 week.

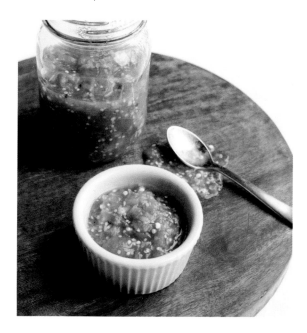

PEPPER-CRUSTED COD
WITH SAMBAL

Sambal is a classic Asian ground chile sauce with a deep smoky flavor highlighted with a touch of fish sauce and dry herbs. It's a super-versatile sauce with medium-high heat. While it's a little fussy to remove the stems and seeds from the dried chiles, it's well worth the effort. **Serves 4**

2 pounds cod steaks or any
    thick white fish
¼ cup all-purpose flour mixed
    with 1 teaspoon coarse salt
    and ½ teaspoon pepper
2 tablespoons olive oil
zest from half a lemon, divided
1 tablespoon whole or coarsely
    ground peppercorns, divided
2 cups mixed bitter baby
    greens (arugula, watercress,
    spinach, or kale)
juice from half a lemon

SAMBAL

2 ounces dried guajillo or
    ancho chiles (5–7 chiles)
¼ cup dried hot Asian
    red chiles
3 cloves garlic, smashed
1 tablespoon minced
    fresh ginger
1 teaspoon sesame oil,
    plus more if needed
juice from 2 limes
½ teaspoon brown sugar
1 teaspoon coarse salt,
    plus more if needed
1 teaspoon fish sauce
½ teaspoon dry cilantro
salt and pepper to taste

TO MAKE THE SAMBAL: Soak the chiles in very hot water for 10 minutes, drain, then remove the stems, skins, and seeds. Combine the chiles with the remaining ingredients in a food processor and pulse until smooth.

TO MAKE THE COD: Lightly dust the cod with the mixture of the flour, salt, and pepper. Gently shake off excess. Heat the olive oil in a heavy skillet over high heat, add the cod, and cook for 3–4 minutes. Sprinkle with half the lemon zest and whole or coarsely ground peppercorns before flipping. Cook an additional 2–3 minutes and sprinkle with remaining lemon zest and peppercorns.

Toss the greens with the lemon juice just before serving. Top with cod and drizzle with the olive oil/peppercorn mixture from the pan. Add a generous spoonful of Sambal to each portion or serve it on the side.

The Sambal will keep in the fridge for at least 1 week.

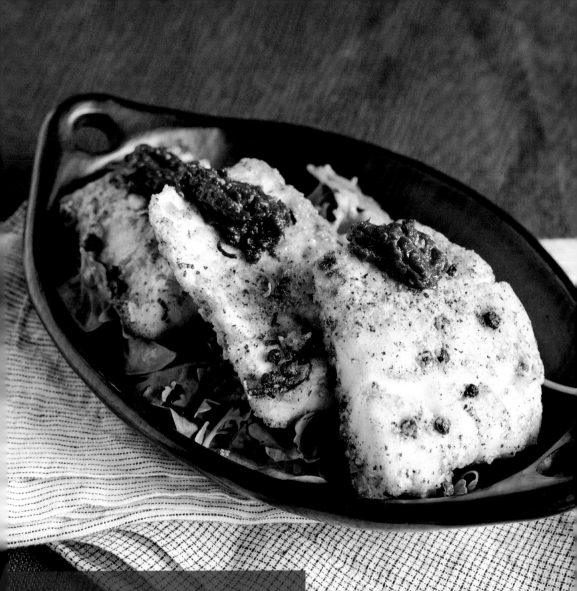

TECHNIQUE

FISH LIKE IT HOT When cooking fish, sear over high heat to get a nice texture and color and lock in all of the flavor. When the heat is not high enough, the fish becomes dry or rubbery.

GINGER BARBECUE SALMON

Pair this salmon with Warm German Potato Salad (see p. 131) or Kabocha Squash Mash (see p. 204), or just keep it easy and serve with grilled bread or rice and a simple salad. If you don't have time to make homemade barbecue sauce, add fresh ginger to a store-bought variety. Plan for about 4–5 ounces per person if you are serving this as a main dish. **Serves 6**

2 pounds salmon
olive oil
coarse salt and pepper

GINGER BARBECUE SAUCE
½ cup Homemade Barbecue
    Sauce (see p. 163)
1 tablespoon minced
    fresh ginger
½ teaspoon coarsely
    ground black pepper

To make the barbecue sauce, stir the fresh ginger and black pepper into the Homemade Barbecue Sauce. Set aside.

Heat the grill to high. Brush fish with olive oil and season with salt and pepper.

Gently lay the salmon skin-side down on the hot grill. Cook about 4–5 minutes, or until the edges begin to char.

Carefully flip over the filet with a metal spatula. Brush with the barbecue sauce and cook about 3–4 minutes, or until the edges begin to char again.

Flip the salmon once more and brush with barbecue sauce again. (Brush the barbecue sauce on after flipping the salmon so you can see the char on it first. After adding the sauce, you want to heat it just long enough to lock in the flavor.)

Cut a little slit in the thickest part of the fish to make sure it's cooked to your liking. Salmon is typically prepared medium rare, or to an internal temperature of 145 degrees.

Note: To prepare the salmon on the stovetop, use a sharp knife to cut the filet into 6 equal portions. Keep the skin on, as it adds flavor during cooking. Cook the salmon starting skin-side down over high heat in a heavy skillet.

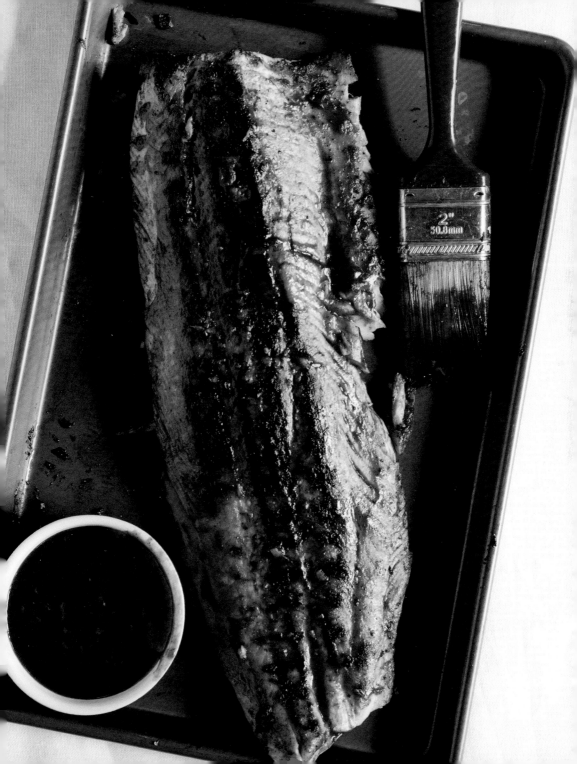

BEYOND BACON

*Pork is a versatile option when you're not in the mood
for chicken. Whatever the cut, pork cooks up tender,
in a pan or on the grill, and plays well with any seasoning.
It's quick and easy to cook—a culinary phenomenon.*

PORK

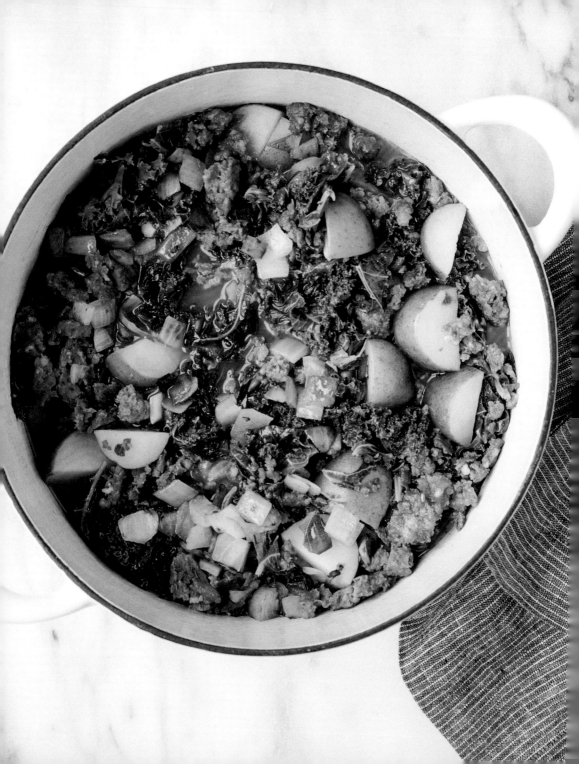

SAUSAGE, POTATO & KALE SOUP

I like to use hot Italian sausage in this soup. As the potato cooks down, the broth thickens, making this a filling soup that offers carbs, leafy greens, and protein—all in one pot! It's proof that simple is also delicious. **Serves 6**

14 ounces bulk Italian sausage
½ cup minced onion
2 cloves garlic, minced
2 pounds small red potatoes, chopped (about 6 cups)
8 cups chicken stock
1 large bunch of kale, stems removed and coarsely chopped
coarse salt and pepper to taste
drizzle of extra-virgin olive oil

Begin by cooking the sausage in a large stockpot over high heat. Continue cooking until the meat is browned and crisp. Drain any excess fat and set aside.

Reduce heat to medium-high and add onion and garlic to the stockpot. Cook a few minutes, stirring frequently, until the onions soften and the garlic is toasted. Add the potatoes and cook a few minutes more to soften slightly before adding the stock.

Partially cover the pot, bring the stock to a rolling boil, and cook the potatoes for 12–15 minutes, or until tender. Add the cooked sausage and stir in the kale and watch for it to turn bright green. When it does, the soup is ready to eat. Season with salt and pepper.

Serve in individual bowls, then top with a drizzle of olive oil to finish.

GRILLED PORK CHOPS WITH KABOCHA SQUASH MASH

To serve up pork chops Tomahawk-style, use a small, sharp knife to score around the bone just above the round of the pork chop and scrape the meat off the top of the bone until clean. Save the scraps for soups, stews, or pasta sauce. I used mine to make Sante Fe Mac 'n' Cheese (see p. 215). The Kabocha Squash Mash is an easy "back burner" recipe that you can have going while you're working on another dish. Any seasonal squash will work: pumpkin, butternut, acorn, etc. Look for a deal and plan for 8 ounces of uncooked squash per person. **Serves 6**

6–8 thick-cut, bone-in
    pork chops (about 3 pounds)
2 tablespoons Basic Grilling
    Salt (see p. 206)
¼ cup olive oil
2 tablespoons Dijon mustard
2 garlic cloves, minced
drizzle of maple syrup
coarse salt

KABOCHA SQUASH MASH

3 pounds kabocha squash
    (acorn or pumpkin also
    work well)
olive oil
coarse salt and pepper to taste
sprinkle of nutmeg
1 Anjou pear, peeled, cored,
    and diced

Let the pork chops warm to room temperature. Heat the oven to 350 degrees.

TO START THE SQUASH: Split the squash lengthwise, scoop out the seeds, and brush the cut sides with olive oil, then sprinkle with salt and pepper. Lay the squash cut-side down on a baking sheet and bake for 30–35 minutes, or until it is soft to the touch.

TO MAKE THE PORK CHOPS: Heat the grill to medium. Brush the pork chops with a little olive oil, then coat liberally with the Basic Grilling Salt.

Heat the oven to 400 degrees. Start the pork chops on the grill, and cook for about 5 minutes on each side to get nice grill marks. Brush with a little olive oil and transfer to the oven to cook for another 15 minutes, or until they reach an internal temperature of 165 degrees. Remove from oven and let the pork chops rest for at least 3 minutes.

TO FINISH THE SQUASH: Scoop the squash out of its skin. Transfer it to a mixing bowl and mash with nutmeg. Gently fold in the diced pears and season to taste with salt and pepper.

Stir together the ¼ cup olive oil, Dijon mustard, and garlic. Place the pork chops on a platter. Top with the dressing and finish with a drizzle of maple syrup and a pinch of coarse salt.

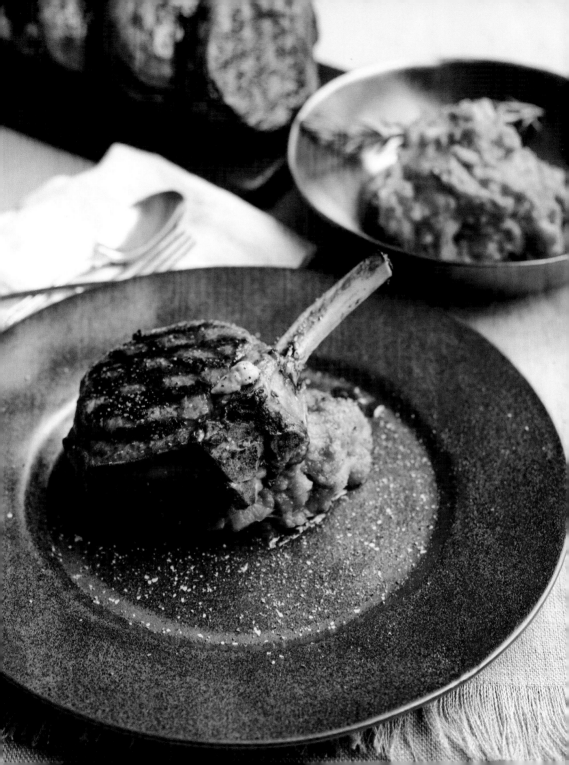

Basic Grilling Salt

This is a versatile grilling salt that holds up to high heat. A touch of sugar gives the meat a nice caramel finish and color. You can use it as a mild rub for chicken and pork.

½ cup coarse salt
2 tablespoons coarse sugar
1 teaspoon ground pepper
½ teaspoon paprika
¼ teaspoon celery seed

Mix together ingredients. Store unused Basic Grilling Salt in an airtight container for future use.

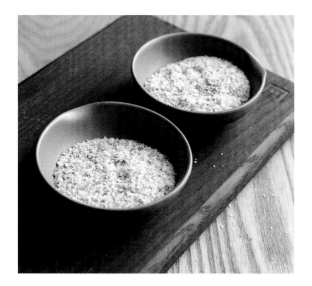

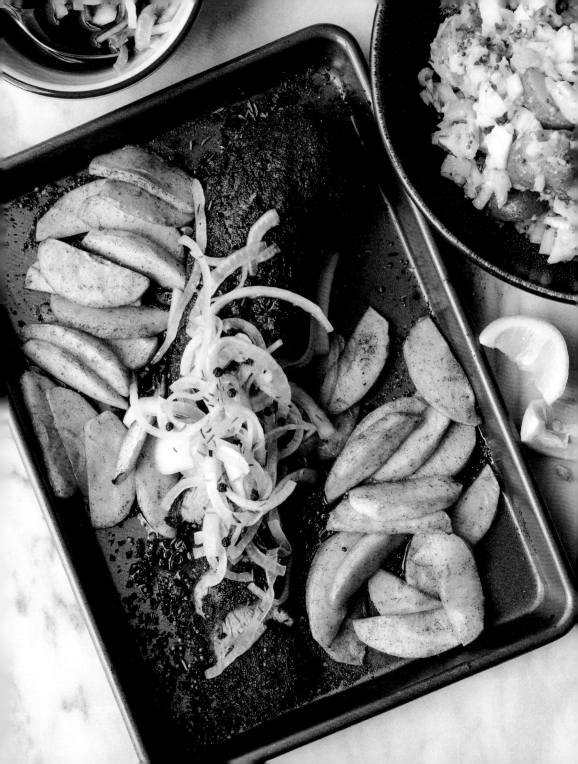

BLACKENED PORK LOIN & PICKLED ONIONS WITH BAKED APPLES

Here's a combination of complex flavors that play well together—the Vindaloo Spice Mix gives the pork rich, bold flavors that are brightened by the pickled onions and balanced with sweet baked apples. Pork loin is great for serving family-style because everyone can help themselves to the portion they want. • Look for baking apples like Granny Smith or Honeycrisp because they give off less moisture. **Serves 6**

2-pound pork loin
up to ¼ cup Vindaloo Spice
    Mix (recipe on p. 209)

BAKED APPLES

3 apples, peeled, cored,
    and cut into thick wedges
1½ teaspoons cinnamon
3 tablespoons sugar
1 tablespoon coconut oil,
    melted, or butter
½ teaspoon salt
zest from half a lemon

PICKLED ONIONS

1 cup thinly sliced white onion
¼ cup red wine vinegar
1 teaspoon whole black
    peppercorns
¼ teaspoon caraway seeds
½ teaspoon coarse salt

Remove the pork loin from the refrigerator and let it come to room temperature.

Rub the meat with the Vindaloo Spice Mix. This is a dry spice rub, meaning the meat will cook without oil, so it might get smoky! You can start it on either the grill or stovetop. Cook over high heat for 3–5 minutes per side to get a good sear on the meat. Once the outside of the meat gets a nice blackened char, remove from heat and transfer to a baking sheet.

Heat the oven to 375 degrees.

Combine the ingredients for the baked apples in a medium bowl and toss to combine. Transfer to the baking sheet along with the pork loin, and bake in the oven for approximately 25–30 minutes, or until the pork is cooked to medium (145 degrees).

TO MAKE THE PICKLED ONIONS: As the pork is cooking, mix together the ingredients for the pickled onions in a small bowl and let sit for at least 5 minutes.

Remove the pork loin from the oven and let it rest before slicing. Top each serving with pickled onions and serve.

ALSO SHOWN WITH WARM GERMAN POTATO SALAD (P. 130).

Vindaloo Spice Mix

Vindaloo is a classic Indian spice mix with robust peppery and bright flavors. At the Little Curry Shop it's one of our most popular items, used to season any meat or vegetable dish with an intense peppery flavor. This is a large batch that will keep for a long time. You can adjust for heat by using less of the spicy items. **Makes about 2½ cups**

1 cup paprika
½ cup whole coriander seeds
½ cup dried whole Asian red chiles
¼ cup chili powder
2 tablespoons whole black peppercorns
1 tablespoon fennel seeds
1½ teaspoons turmeric
1½ teaspoons cumin seeds
1½ teaspoons cayenne pepper
1½ teaspoons coarse salt
1 teaspoon dry cilantro
2 teaspoons mango powder (optional)

Toast all of the ingredients in a dry sauté pan over medium-high heat until the larger seeds are golden and there is a warm fragrance coming from the pan. Do not let it smoke! Remove from heat, let cool, then grind thoroughly in a blender or spice mill until you have a coarse powder.

Note: The key ingredients in vindaloo are coriander, paprika, salt, pepper, and heat. Everything else is basically optional. The mango powder adds tartness, but if you can't get mango powder you can simply add some vinegar or lemon juice when finishing your dish.

FLASH PICKLING

Similar to a fresh slaw, this is another way to add a layer of bright flavor to a heavy dish or protein. Letting fresh vegetables sit in vinegar and salt softens the texture and the bite.

The traditional method for flash pickling requires that you boil all of your ingredients. Since we are simply finishing our dish rather than storing these ingredients for an extended period of time, you can skip that step. Simply let the crunchy base marinate in the vinegar for 5–10 minutes or until the vegetables soften up a little.

Start with thin-sliced, flavorful, crunchy vegetables:

onions, radishes, fennel, leeks

Add vinegar. Use lighter vinegars to preserve the color of your vegetables and bring a light, bright flavor. Darker vinegars will add color and deeper flavor.

Aged vinegars generally have a softer, more complex flavor. Less expensive varieties tend to be more harsh, but if you find the flavor is too strong, just add a splash of water.

Finish it off with seasoning to taste:

capers, green peppercorns, coarse salt, coarse sugar

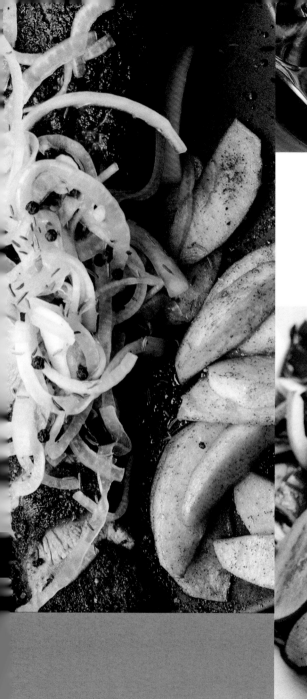
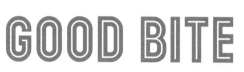

GOOD BITE

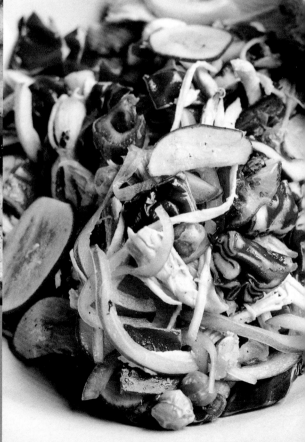

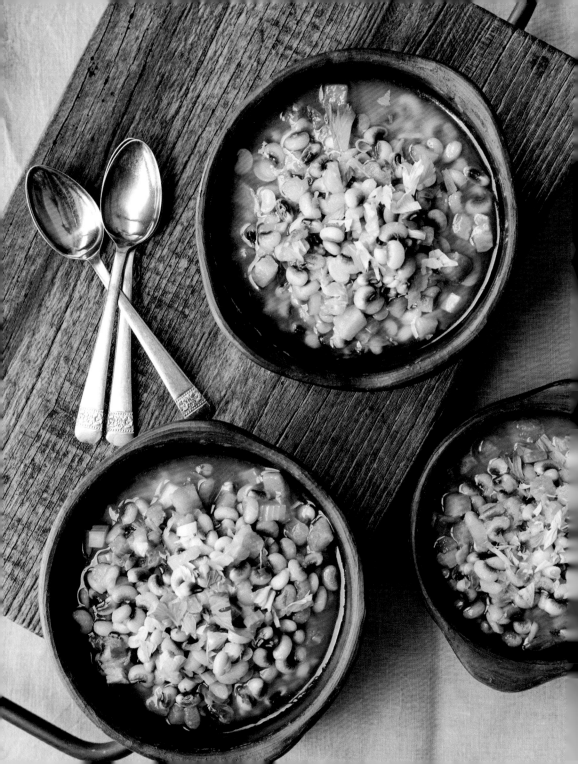

STEWED BLACK-EYED PEAS WITH SALT PORK

Here's a little bowl of Americana. I use frozen black-eyed peas because they cook up in 10 minutes and keep their texture better than dry or canned beans because they are picked fresh and immediately frozen. Canned beans won't work in this recipe, so don't waste your time trying. Do try out the salt pork—it's affordable and delicious in this dish. **Serves 6**

8 ounces salt pork or
   thick-cut bacon, diced
   into quarter-inch cubes
1 cup minced onion
2 cloves garlic, minced
1½ cups low-sodium
   chicken stock
½ cup chopped celery
1 pound frozen or fresh-cooked
   black-eyed peas

ON TOP
extra-virgin olive oil
chopped celery leaves
lemon juice to taste
freshly grated Parmesan
chopped fresh oregano
   (optional)

Add the salt pork or bacon to a heavy pot over medium-high heat and cook about 15 minutes, or until crisp. (With salt pork be patient; it can take a while to get it right, but it's worth the wait.) Tip the pan to spoon off the excess fat. Add the onion and garlic and cook until the onions are translucent, about 2–3 minutes. Add the stock and stir. Bring to a low rolling boil.

Lower the heat to medium. Add in the celery and black-eyed peas (no need to thaw) and simmer for 10–15 minutes until heated through. The beans and celery will brighten as they heat up.

Taste. If the pork makes the dish too salty, drizzle with olive oil before serving. Ladle into individual bowls and finish with celery leaves, fresh lemon juice, a sprinkle of grated Parmesan, and oregano, if desired.

TRY THIS WITH CATFISH PICCATA (P. 183) FOR SOME SOUTHERN COMFORT FOOD.

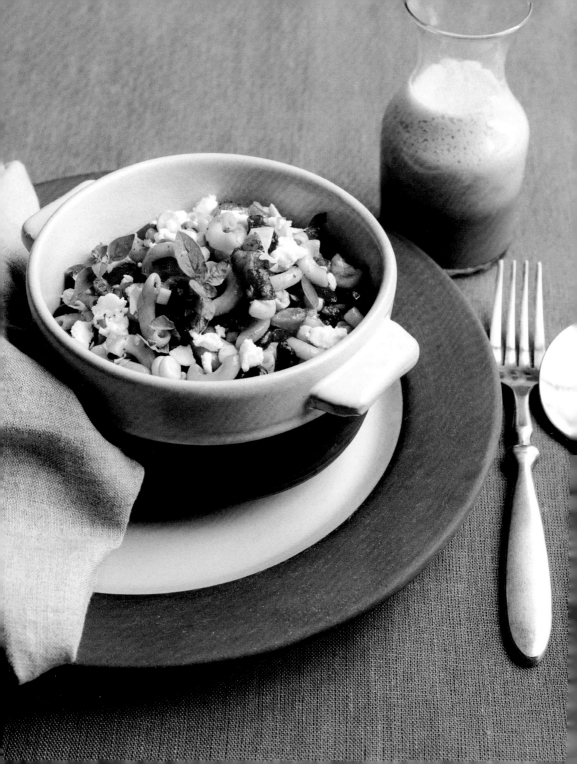

SANTA FE
MAC 'N' CHEESE

This is a great way to use up leftover meat or scraps in a tasty pasta dish—we used the trimmings from our Grilled Pork Chops (see p. 204). Shredded meat also works well, whether pork or rotisserie chicken. To really bring the bright, intense Santa Fe flavors to life, I blitz it with some fresh hot sauce. There's no oil to hold back the heat of the jalapeños in this sauce, so start with a small drizzle. **Serves 4**

8 ounces uncooked small pasta
    (elbow, farfalle, or your
    favorite shape)
1 tablespoon olive oil
8 ounces uncooked chicken
    or pork, chopped,
    or 2 cups cooked meat
½ cup diced red onion
1 teaspoon Mexican seasoning
    (chili powder and cumin)
1 15-ounce can black beans or
    2 cups cooked beans
1 cup small tomatoes, cut in
    half lengthwise
1 ear of fresh sweet corn,
    kernels cut off the cob,
    or 1 cup frozen sweet corn
1 jalapeño, diced
¼ cup crumbled farmer cheese,
    queso fresco, or any soft,
    fresh milk cheese
¼ cup fresh herbs
    (oregano, cilantro, or sage)

**FRESH JALAPEÑO
HOT SAUCE**
3 jalapeños, stems removed
½ cup white vinegar, divided
1 teaspoon coarse salt

Bring a large pot of salted water to a boil and prepare the pasta as directed on the package. Drain the pasta and set it aside.

In a sauté pan over medium-high heat, warm the olive oil. Add the meat and cook 4–5 minutes until golden brown. (If you are using leftover meat, simply heat it.) Add the red onion and Mexican seasoning and stir to combine. Cook 3–4 minutes, until the onions are translucent.

If using canned beans, drain and rinse them. Fold the black beans and cooked pasta into the meat mixture and heat. Remove from heat and add the remaining ingredients—tomatoes, corn, jalapeño, crumbled cheese, and fresh herbs.

TO MAKE THE HOT SAUCE: Combine the jalapeños, half of the vinegar, and salt in a blender and pulse to combine, then slowly pour in the remaining vinegar and blend long enough to purée the jalapeños. You will get some foam on top, and the sauce will separate if it sits. Just give it a stir before serving.

Serve the pasta in individual bowls with a drizzle of hot sauce.

ROAST PORK LOIN WITH PEACH GLAZE & WHITE BEANS

This pork is great for sandwiches or wraps, or you can serve it on top of a warm white bean salad with fresh chopped herbs. Don't be intimidated by the fancy presentation. A rustic presentation with thick-cut slices will taste equally amazing. **Serves 6**

2-pound pork loin
2 tablespoons Basic Grilling
 Salt (see p. 206)
1 tablespoon olive oil
¼ cup chunky peach preserves,
 divided

WHITE BEANS

2 cups uncooked butter beans
 or large lima beans
4 cups water or stock
¼ cup minced fresh parsley
1 garlic clove, sliced thin
1 heaping tablespoon minced
 fresh chives
1 tablespoon extra-virgin
 olive oil
juice from 1 lemon
½ teaspoon coarse salt
¼ teaspoon pepper
2 tablespoons maple syrup
⅛ teaspoon Ghost Pepper
 Salt Mix (see p. 84)

TO START THE BEANS: Rinse and sort the beans to remove any debris or discolored beans. Cover with cold water and let soak in the fridge for at least 1 hour. Large beans work best if soaked just a couple of hours before cooking. Drain the water.

Place the beans and salted water or stock in a medium stockpot. Make sure the liquid covers the beans. Bring to a rolling boil then reduce heat to low and let simmer for 1 hour, or until tender.

Heat the oven to 375 degrees.

TO MAKE THE PORK: Season the pork loin with grilling salt. (If you don't have any on hand, season with coarse salt and pepper and a sprinkle of celery salt.)

In an oven-safe sauté pan over high heat, heat the olive oil and sear the loin until you have a nice even brown color all around.

Brush the pork loin with 3 tablespoons peach preserves and bake in the oven for 25–30 minutes, or until the temperature of the meat reaches 145 degrees. Remove and let rest for about 5 minutes.

TO FINISH THE BEANS: Once the beans are finished cooking, drain and rinse under cool water. In a mixing bowl, combine parsley, garlic, chives, olive oil, lemon juice, salt, and pepper and gently fold in the cooked beans. Finish with maple syrup and Ghost Pepper Salt Mix.

Add another spoonful of preserves to the pork loin before serving, then slice thin with a sharp knife.

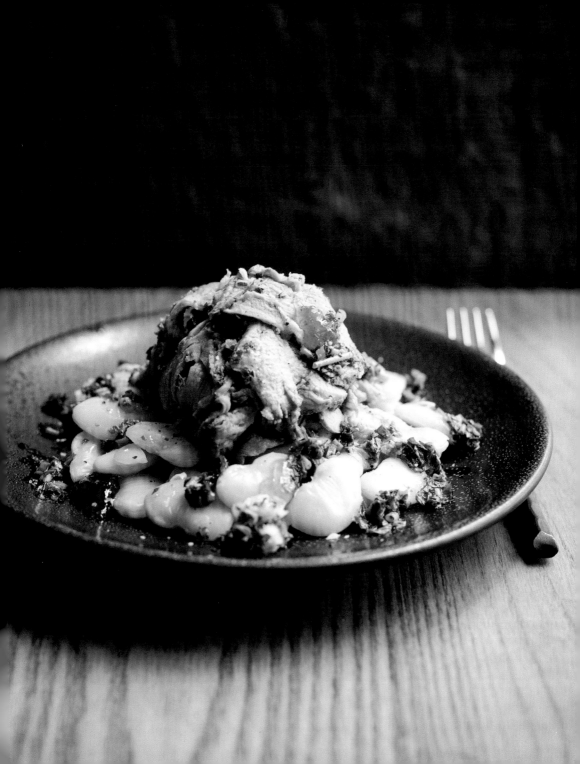

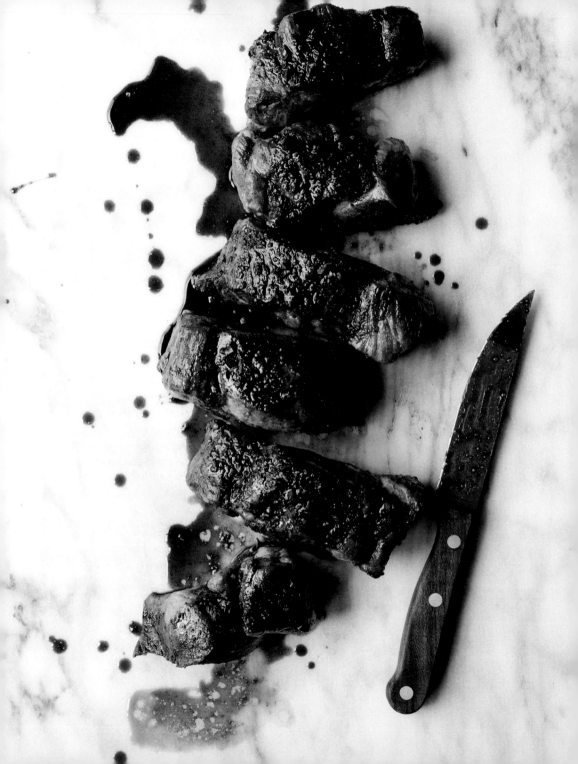

COUNTRY-STYLE HOISIN RIBS

Ribs are a quintessential family-style meal. Sit back and watch everyone throwing elbows and reaching in for more. A homemade sauce makes the experience (and the ribs) even better! Hoisin sauce is the Asian spin on spicy-sweet barbecue sauce. Black bean paste is a common ingredient, but it can be very salty and difficult to find. I opted to use red miso instead, which you can then use to make our other Asian-inspired recipes. **Serves 6**

4 pounds country-style or
    baby back pork ribs
2 tablespoons Basic Grilling
    Salt (see p. 206) or
    1 tablespoon coarse salt
    and 1 teaspoon pepper

HOISIN SAUCE
1 teaspoon sesame oil
2 teaspoons minced
    fresh ginger
1 clove garlic, minced
1 tablespoon minced jalapeño
1 tablespoon Chinese
    five-spice powder
½ cup low-sodium soy sauce
    or liquid aminos
½ cup packed brown sugar
2 tablespoons molasses
2 tablespoons tahini
    (sesame paste)
1 teaspoon miso, plus additional
    to taste
2 tablespoons rice wine vinegar

Heat the oven to 375 degrees.

Trim any excess fat off of the ribs. Rub with grilling salt or a mixture of coarse salt and pepper. Place the ribs on a baking sheet in the middle rack of the oven and bake for 45 minutes. While the ribs are baking, start the Hoisin Sauce.

TO MAKE THE HOISIN: Add the sesame oil to a small saucepan over medium heat. Add the ginger, garlic, and jalapeño, and stir until they start to brown. Then add the Chinese five-spice, stirring to incorporate. Whisk in the remaining ingredients and cover the pan to bring the mixture to a low rolling boil. Reduce heat to low and let the sauce simmer until thick, about 10 minutes. Let cool. Adjust sauce to taste with additional red miso. Reserve half of the sauce in a serving bowl and use the other half for brushing on the ribs during cooking.

After 45 minutes, remove the ribs from the oven and brush generously with Hoisin Sauce. Flip and brush again with the sauce. Return the pan to the oven and bake for another 30–45 minutes, or until fork-tender and falling off the bone. It can take up to 2 hours total to bake the ribs. Continue brushing with the Hoisin Sauce every 30 minutes or so until the ribs are done. Serve with leftover sauce . . . and napkins.

WHILE THE RIBS ARE COOKING MAKE SOME SWEET POTATO-STUFFED WONTON SOUP (P. 121).

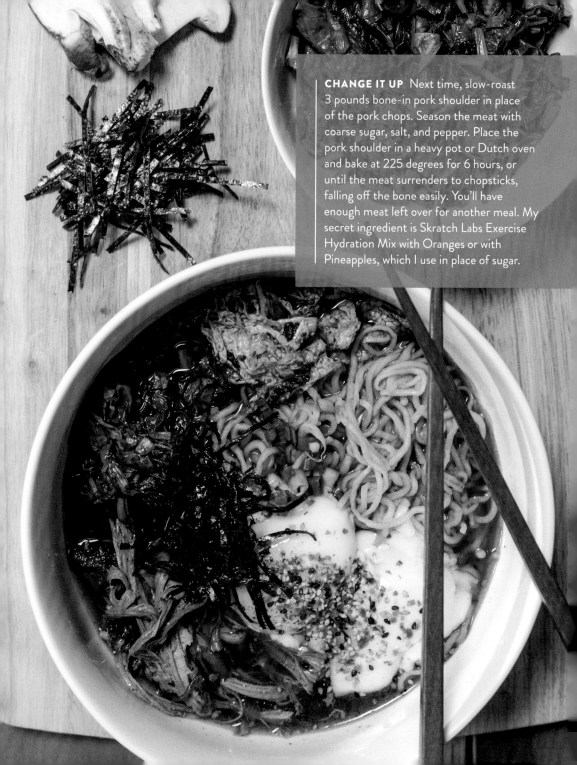

CHANGE IT UP Next time, slow-roast 3 pounds bone-in pork shoulder in place of the pork chops. Season the meat with coarse sugar, salt, and pepper. Place the pork shoulder in a heavy pot or Dutch oven and bake at 225 degrees for 6 hours, or until the meat surrenders to chopsticks, falling off the bone easily. You'll have enough meat left over for another meal. My secret ingredient is Skratch Labs Exercise Hydration Mix with Oranges or with Pineapples, which I use in place of sugar.

ALLEN'S RAMEN

Ramen is the epitome of comfort food for me. But making traditional ramen from scratch takes a lot of time and patience. This recipe is a hybrid of tradition and convenience. There are shortcuts that can make this recipe even easier, like using store-bought noodles and stock. Still, there's nothing like homemade noodles and the depth of flavor that develops when you take the time to make your own stock and broth. **Serves 4**

1 pound bone-in pork chops
1 tablespoon coarse sugar
1 tablespoon coarse salt
1 teaspoon pepper
4 eggs
1 bunch spinach, chopped
1 cup frozen corn (optional)
1 cup frozen peas (optional)

QUICK BROTH

8 cups chicken stock or
   homemade Beef Bone
   Stock (p. 98)
1 piece kombu seaweed
2 cups bonita fish flakes

SHOYU BASE

1 cup shoyu (Japanese
   soy sauce)
¼ cup coarse sugar
¼ cup mirin (rice cooking wine)

NOODLES

Ramen Noodles (see p. 224)
   or 4 servings of frozen
   ramen noodles

ON TOP

1 bunch diced green onions
½ cup dried seaweed
salt and pepper to taste

Note: Sun Noodle makes authentic ramen noodles that can be found in the frozen food section of many Chinese or Korean supermarkets (www.sunnoodle.com).

TO MAKE THE QUICK BROTH: In a stockpot, combine the ingredients and simmer for about 30 minutes.

Rub the pork chops with sugar, salt, and pepper and panfry over medium heat for about 4–5 minutes on each side, or until cooked to medium (internal temperature of 145 degrees). Let rest for 30 minutes, then slice and set aside.

TO MAKE THE SHOYU BASE: In a separate small pot, combine the ingredients and stir over medium heat until the sugar is completely dissolved.

To make the ramen soup, remove kombu and strain bonita flakes from the Quick Broth. Use the Shoyu Base to season your broth, adding ½ cup at a time to taste. When the ramen broth (soup base) is seasoned to your liking, cover and let simmer in the stockpot over low heat as you prepare the other components.

Soft-boil eggs for 5 minutes, then allow to cool before peeling. (You can also poach them: Fill a shallow medium saucepan halfway with water and add a pinch of salt. Bring to a rolling boil and then crack the eggs into a small bowl one at a time and gently slide them into the boiling water. Cook for 5–6 minutes, or until the eggs are fully white. Drain with a slotted spoon and set aside.)

(recipe continues)

Sauté spinach with corn and peas, if using, in pan over medium-high heat for about 3–4 minutes, or until the spinach wilts, then set aside.

Evenly distribute grilled meat, cooked eggs, and sautéed vegetables into individual bowls just before boiling the ramen noodles.

Add ramen noodles to boiling salted water in as large of a pot as you have. Boil noodles for 3–4 minutes or until tender but still chewy and firm. It's easiest to cook a single serving of noodles in a wire ramen basket or strainer to keep each serving separate. After cooking, immediately divide noodles among individual bowls.

Bring soup base back up to a low boil, then ladle soup into individual bowls. Garnish with green onions and dried seaweed, and add salt and pepper to taste.

Slow Broth

I typically start this on a Saturday afternoon and cook it overnight. You start by boiling in the flavor of the kombu seaweed and bonita flakes, then cook the chicken for a couple of hours, then add the pork bones and let simmer overnight with the onions and mushrooms.

6 quarts water
2 pieces kombu seaweed
4 cups bonita fish flakes
1 whole chicken
2 pounds pork bones
3–4 whole onions, quartered
8 ounces shitake mushrooms

Fill a 12-quart stockpot with water. Add kombu seaweed and boil for about 30 minutes. Remove kombu and add bonita flakes. Let them boil for 15 minutes before removing with a strainer.

Add the whole chicken and let boil for about 2–3 hours. Remove chicken.

Add about 2 pounds of assorted pork bones and let simmer overnight with onions, mushrooms, and any other vegetables you might have on hand. As the water boils off, more will need to be added so that you will end up with 6 quarts of broth.

Remove bones and strain the broth. Store using 8 cups of broth at a time with Shoyu Base (in place of Quick Broth) to create ramen soup.

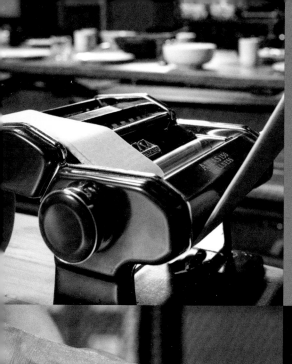

There's a Chinese tradition of having noodles on your birthday. As the superstition goes, the longer the noodle is, the longer your life will be. This is why Allen makes his from scratch.

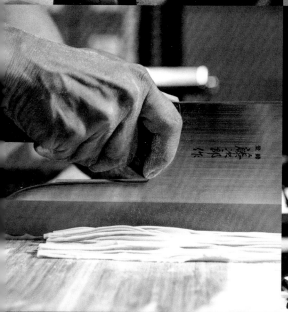

MAKE IT SPECIAL

RAMEN NOODLES

Although instant ramen noodles are convenient and tasty, because they're flash-fried they have a higher fat content, they don't have the same texture as fresh or frozen noodles, and they often contain preservatives such as propylene glycol. Making your own ramen noodles is a relatively simple and fun option, and with a little practice and experimentation homemade noodles can rival store-bought options. Just make sure you let the dough rest so the gluten can form, and always boil your ramen noodles in as large of a pot as possible to help wash away the excess starch that can make the noodles bitter and slimy.

4 cups pastry or bread flour
½ teaspoon sodium carbonate
just under 1 cup water at room temperature

Note: *Sodium carbonate is hard to find in stores but is readily available online. You can also make it by heating baking soda in the oven at 300 degrees for about 30 minutes. This will cook off H_2O, converting sodium bicarbonate to sodium carbonate. Adding sodium carbonate to the ramen dough makes the noodles more alkaline, which helps them hold up in hot broth.*

1

In a stand mixer with a dough hook, mix ingredients at medium speed for 2–3 minutes until dough forms. If dough doesn't form in that time, add 1 teaspoon of water at a time until dough holds together. Continue kneading for 10 minutes in stand mixer or on a lightly floured work surface for 10 minutes or until it is smooth and elastic. Shape into a ball and let it rest in the fridge for about 2 hours.

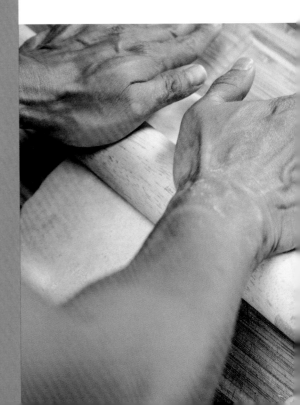

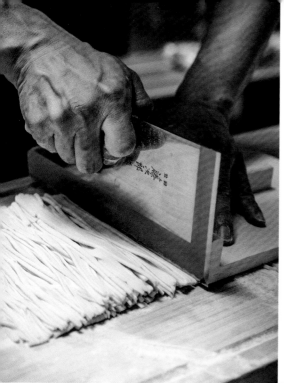

3

Use the largest pot you have to cook no more than 2 servings of noodles at a time in salted boiling water. Place the noodles in a wire basket or strainer and lower into the water for 3–4 minutes, or until texture is firm and slightly chewy.

2

Roll out the dough as thinly as possible. Fold dough back on itself and repeat process 3–4 times to work gluten. After rolling out a final time, use a large knife and carefully cut dough into thin noodles. (You can also use a pasta maker to roll out and cut the noodles.) Lightly dust with flour to keep noodles from sticking together. Separate noodles into 4 equal servings.

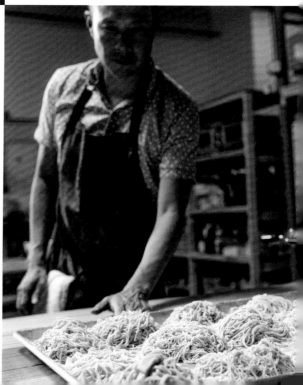

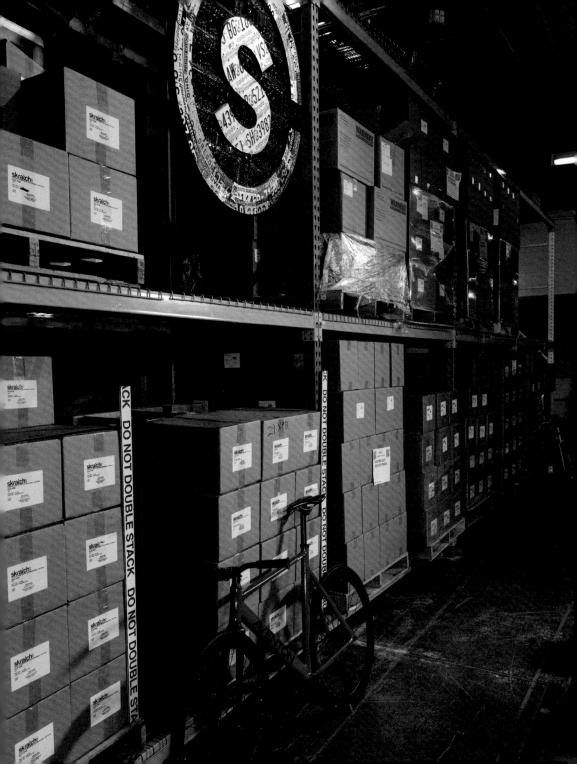

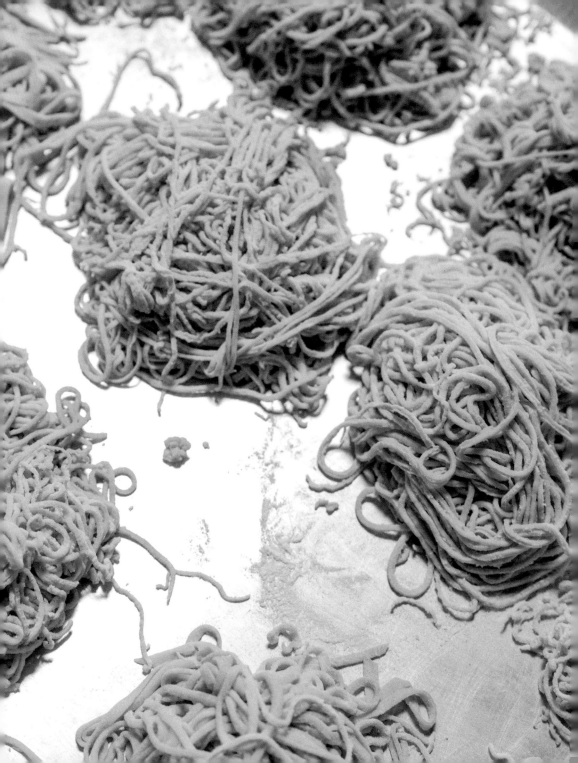

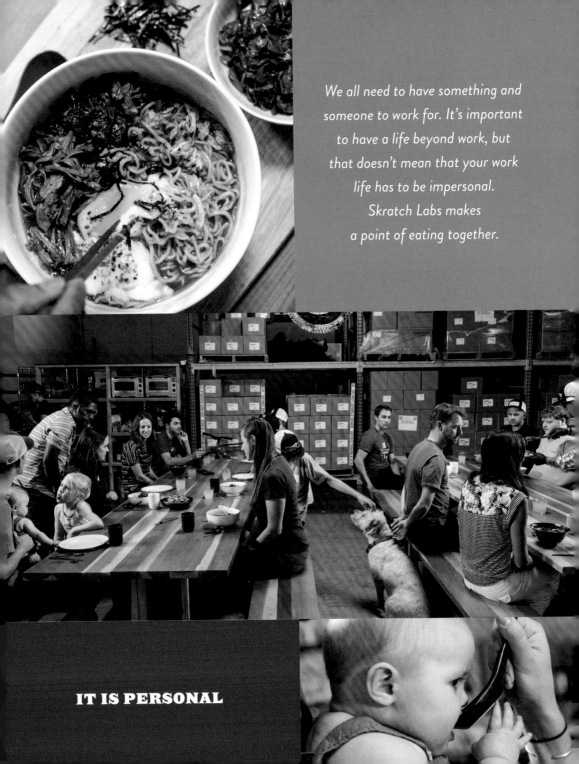

We all need to have something and someone to work for. It's important to have a life beyond work, but that doesn't mean that your work life has to be impersonal. Skratch Labs makes a point of eating together.

IT IS PERSONAL

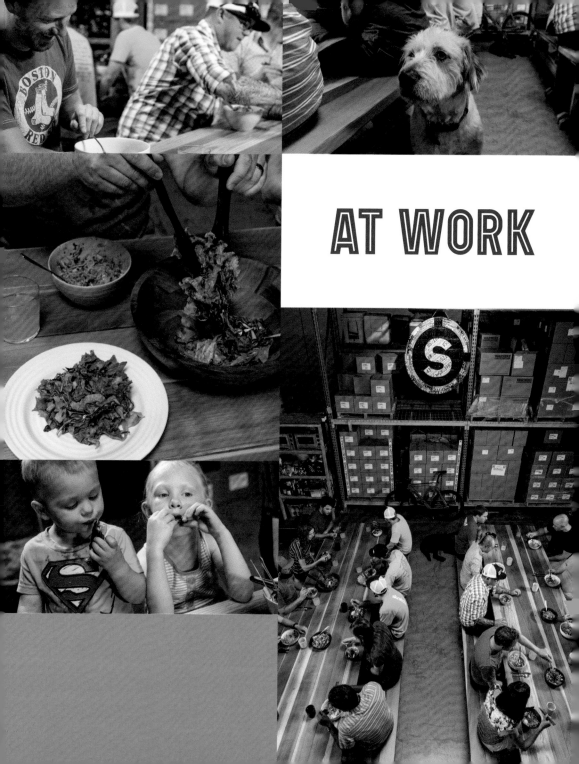

AT WORK

A REAL TREAT

Red meat is indulgent. We consider any of these meats to be a treat. Eating red meat less often will save you money while also helping our planet. And the occasional steak will taste even better.

BEEF
LAMB
BISON

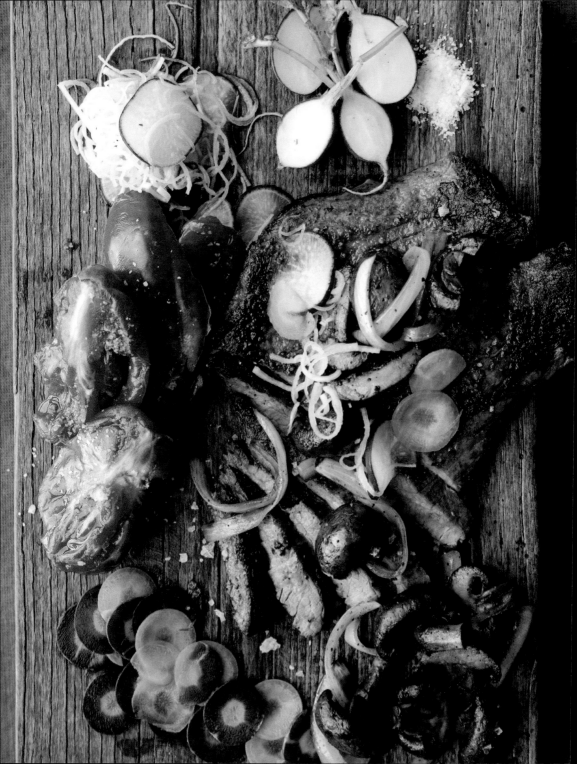

FLANK STEAK WITH TORN HEIRLOOM TOMATOES

A little meat goes a long way if you serve it up family-style with some cooked grains or thick-cut rustic bread. Add as many different-colored fresh-chopped vegetables to the spread as you can, then punch up the flavor with this simple Radish & Leek Slaw. **Serves 6**

2 pounds flank steak
1 tablespoon coarse salt
½ teaspoon pepper
sprinkle of coarse sugar
1 tablespoon olive oil
8 ounces baby portabellas
   or small brown mushrooms,
   sliced
¼ onion, thinly sliced
3–4 heirloom tomatoes,
   destemmed and pulled
   into pieces
drizzle of extra-virgin olive oil
coarse salt to taste
splash of red wine vinegar
1 cup chopped carrots

RADISH & LEEK SLAW

1 small bunch radishes,
   sliced into thin rounds
1 leek, white part only,
   rinsed and sliced thin
1 tablespoon red wine vinegar
juice from 1 lemon
1 teaspoon coarse salt
sprinkle of coarse sugar

Let the steak come to room temperature. Trim off any excess fat and silver parts, then season with salt and pepper and a sprinkle of coarse sugar.

Heat the olive oil in a large sauté pan over high heat, then sear the steak for 4–5 minutes on each side to cook to medium.

TO MAKE THE SLAW: While the meat is finishing up, wash and prepare the radishes and leeks. Mix them together in a small bowl with the red wine vinegar, lemon juice, salt, and sugar.

TO FINISH THE DISH: When the steak is done cooking, remove it from heat and let it rest for just a few minutes while you cook the sliced mushrooms and onions in the same pan—just long enough for the mushrooms to get some color and the onions to soften and become translucent, about 3 minutes over high heat.

Place the heirloom tomatoes in a large bowl and add a drizzle of olive oil, coarse salt, and a splash of red wine vinegar. Repeat with the carrots.

Slice the meat across the grain, then serve on a large platter or cutting board surrounded with the sautéed mushrooms, garden vegetables, and slaw.

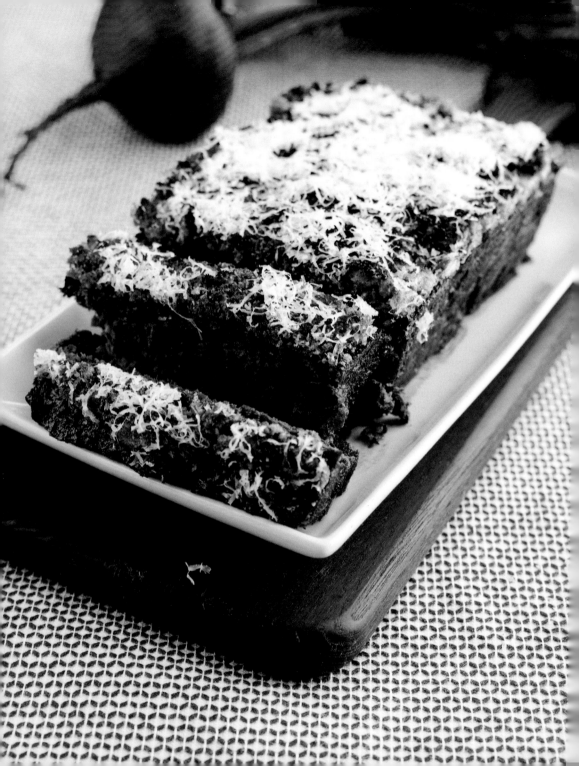

BEEF & BEET MEATLOAF

Our friends affectionately refer to this as "beetloaf"—the beets are spectacularly sweet and earthy, taking this meatloaf to a whole new level. Try it as a sandwich or alongside a fresh green salad. **Serves 6**

1 pound ground beef
1 cup red beets, peeled and shredded
1 cup bread crumbs (gluten-free will work)
2 eggs, lightly beaten
½ cup minced onion
1 tablespoon minced garlic
1 tablespoon soy sauce
1 tablespoon ketchup or Homemade Barbecue Sauce (see p. 163)
1 tablespoon of your favorite Italian seasoning
1 teaspoon coarse salt

ON TOP
1 cup bread crumbs
1 tablespoon olive oil
½ cup freshly grated Parmesan, loosely packed

Heat the oven to 375 degrees. Lightly coat a 5 × 9–inch loaf pan with nonstick cooking spray.

Put all of the meatloaf ingredients into a large mixing bowl and work the mixture with your hands until everything is incorporated. Transfer the beef mixture into the prepared loaf pan, smoothing the top of the loaf as you fill the pan, and put it in the oven to bake for 40 minutes.

While the meatloaf is baking, stir together the topping ingredients. Sprinkle this bread crumb mixture on top of the meatloaf after it has cooked for 40 minutes. (You can also brush on more ketchup or barbecue sauce at this point, if desired.) Return the loaf to the top rack of the oven.

Bake for another 10–15 minutes. The meat will shrink slightly as it cooks, pulling away from the edge of the pan. Remove from oven and let cool for a moment before slicing and serving.

THE MIXED BEAN CURRY (P. 259) MAKES A FLAVORFUL SIDE TO THIS MEATLOAF.

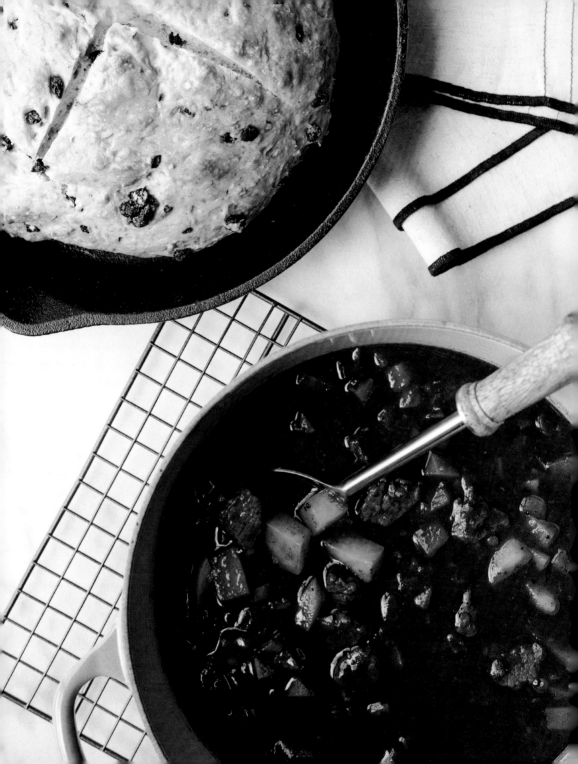

IRISH LAMB STEW WITH GUINNESS & SODA BREAD

The combination of lamb and Guinness makes a smoky stew with nice earthy flavors. Fingerling potatoes hold up well in this dish because they are less starchy, but you can use whatever you have on hand. **Serves 8**

2 pounds lamb, cubed
¼ cup flour mixed with
    1 teaspoon salt and
    ½ teaspoon pepper
olive oil
1 cup diced onion
1 cup diced carrots
1 cup diced celery
1 tablespoon malt vinegar
1 tablespoon Worcestershire
    sauce
1 pound coarsely chopped
    potatoes (about 3 cups)
1 cup canned crushed tomatoes
    or about 2 cups chopped
    fresh tomatoes
1 12-ounce bottle of Guinness
4 cups beef stock
salt and pepper to taste

SODA BREAD
4 cups all-purpose flour
1 teaspoon caraway seeds
1 cup currants or raisins
1 teaspoon baking soda
1 teaspoon salt
1¾ cups buttermilk
1 egg
1 egg plus 1 tablespoon water,
    lightly beaten
sprinkle of coarse sugar

TO MAKE THE STEW: Lightly dust the lamb with the mixture of flour, salt, and pepper.

In a large stockpot over high heat, warm just enough olive oil to coat the bottom of the pan. Add the lamb, onions, carrots, and celery and cook until the meat browns, about 8–10 minutes.

Deglaze the bottom of the pan with the malt vinegar and Worcestershire sauce by scraping it with a wooden spoon. Then add the potatoes and crushed tomatoes and stir until well combined.

Add the Guinness and the beef stock. Bring to a low rolling boil, then reduce the heat to low and simmer, covered, for 45 minutes, or until the lamb is good and tender. Before serving, season the stew to taste with salt and pepper.

While the stew is cooking, make the Soda Bread.

TO MAKE SODA BREAD: Heat the oven to 350 degrees.

Lightly coat an 8-inch round pan with nonstick cooking spray or use a seasoned cast-iron pan close to the same size. (Note that with a cast-iron pan cooking time might be 5–10 minutes less.)

Start by mixing together the flour, caraway seeds, currants or raisins, baking soda, and salt in a large bowl until well combined. In a large liquid measuring cup, combine the buttermilk and egg, and lightly whisk.

(recipe continues)

Pour the wet ingredients into the flour mixture and stir together until all of the flour is incorporated. You will have a thick, sticky dough. Lightly knead the dough on a floured surface, then shape it into a ball.

Transfer the dough into the greased pan and use a sharp knife to cut an X in the top of the loaf. As the loaf bakes, the X will split open a bit more. Bake for 35 minutes, then brush the top of the soda bread with the egg wash and sprinkle with coarse sugar. Bake an additional 10 minutes, or until you have a nice golden brown crust.

Remove the bread from the oven and place it on a rack to cool. Serve soda bread while it is still slightly warm, crusty on the outside and soft and chewy inside.

Note: For a dairy-free soda bread, instead of using buttermilk add 2 tablespoons of lemon juice to 1¾ cups almond or soy milk and let sit for five minutes.

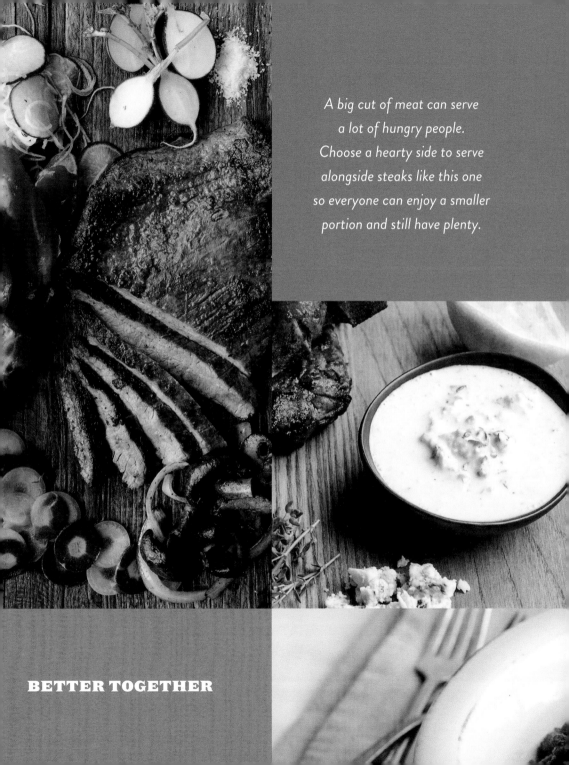

*A big cut of meat can serve
a lot of hungry people.
Choose a hearty side to serve
alongside steaks like this one
so everyone can enjoy a smaller
portion and still have plenty.*

BETTER TOGETHER

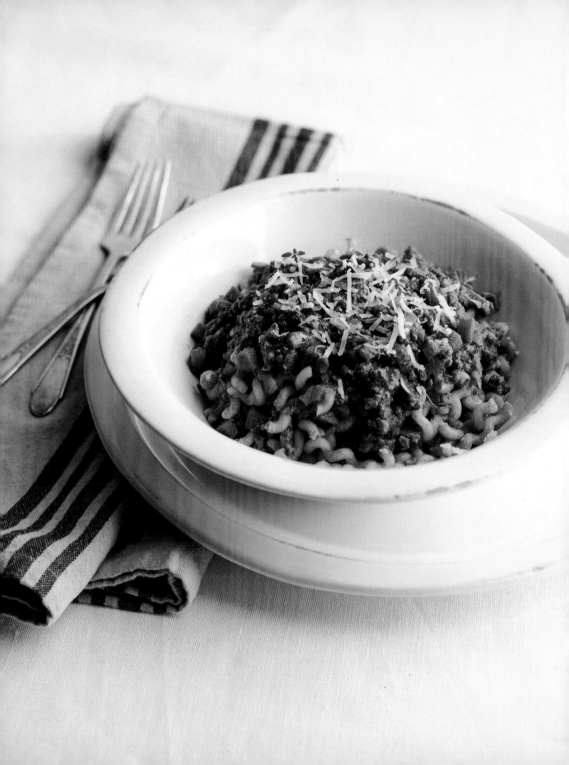

MAC 'N' CHEESE BOLOGNESE

Professional cycling teams are served plenty of boiled chicken and overcooked spaghetti when they are traveling from race to race and eating hotel fare. At the 2015 Tour of California, Mark Cavendish requested that we make him some Bolognese. Our team made him a special batch, and he went on to win that day's stage . . . just saying. **Serves 6**

8 ounces uncooked elbow macaroni or curly noodles
1 cup minced bacon
1 pound ground beef
½ cup minced onion
½ cup finely diced carrots
½ cup minced celery
2 cloves minced garlic
½ cup tomato paste
1 cup dry white wine
1 cup whole milk
1 large tomato, diced
2 tablespoons chopped fresh herbs (parsley, thyme, basil, or a mixture)
coarse salt and pepper to taste
freshly grated Parmesan

Bring a large pot of salted water to a boil and prepare the pasta as directed on the package. Drain the pasta and set aside.

Brown the bacon in a heavy pot over medium-high heat until crisp. Add the ground beef and continue to cook until browned. Add the onion, carrots, celery, and garlic, and cook until the carrots are tender, about 5–6 minutes. Drain any excess fat from the pan.

Add the tomato paste and use a wooden spoon to fully incorporate it, scraping the bottom of the pan. Turn the heat down to medium and add the white wine, cooking about 5 minutes to reduce the liquid and let the flavors meld. Turn the heat off and quickly stir in the milk until well combined.

Finish with the diced tomato and fresh herbs, and season with salt and pepper to taste. Toss with pasta and garnish with Parmesan.

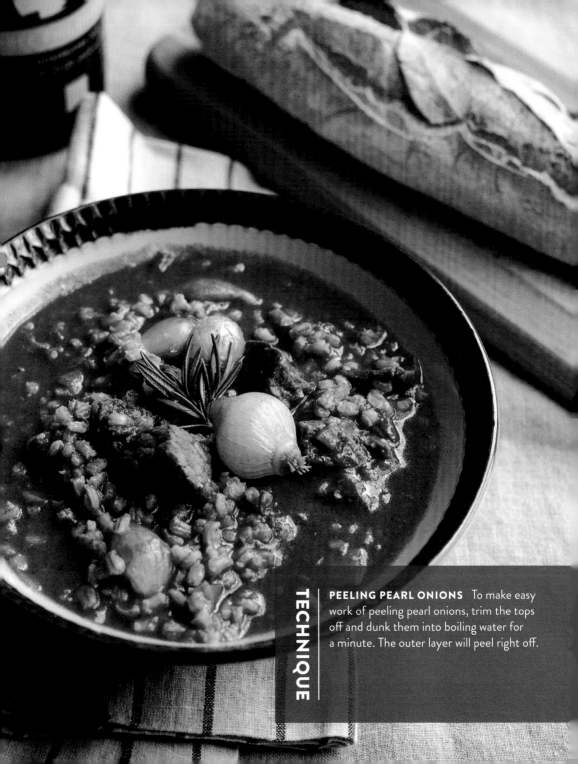

TECHNIQUE

PEELING PEARL ONIONS To make easy work of peeling pearl onions, trim the tops off and dunk them into boiling water for a minute. The outer layer will peel right off.

BISON STEW WITH BARLEY & BELGIAN BEER

You can use beef, bison, or any lean red meat to make this hearty stew. Use our shortcut to peel pearled onions and enjoy the sweet flavor they add. If you don't have the patience for that, dice up some yellow onions and spend your time finding a good Belgian beer instead. **Serves 8**

2 pounds bison stew meat
¼ cup all-purpose flour mixed
   with 1 teaspoon coarse salt
   and ½ teaspoon pepper
2 tablespoons olive oil
10 ounces pearl onions or
   1 cup diced yellow onion
1 cup diced carrots
½ cup tomato paste
1 teaspoon celery salt or
   Old Bay seasoning
1 cup uncooked barley
4 cups beef stock
1 12-oz. bottle of Abbey ale
   (divided)

Lightly dust the stew meat with the mixture of flour, coarse salt, and pepper. Shake gently to remove extra flour. Lightly coat the bottom of a large stockpot with olive oil and bring to high heat. Add the stew meat, scraping the bottom of the pan as you brown the meat. (If you are using yellow onions in place of pearl onions, add them now and cook until translucent.) Cook until the meat has an even color on all sides, about 5–7 minutes. Add the carrots and cook until they begin to soften, about 3 minutes.

Next add the tomato paste and celery salt or Old Bay seasoning and continue scraping the bottom of the pan to keep the mixture from sticking, stirring for 1–2 minutes more. Stir in the barley, letting the heat toast it slightly, then add the stock and half of the Abbey ale. Let simmer at a medium rolling boil, covered, for 30 minutes.

If using pearl onions, add them now and half of the beer and let simmer another 30 minutes or until the bison is tender. If the opened beer has survived the wait, stir in the rest of it right before serving.

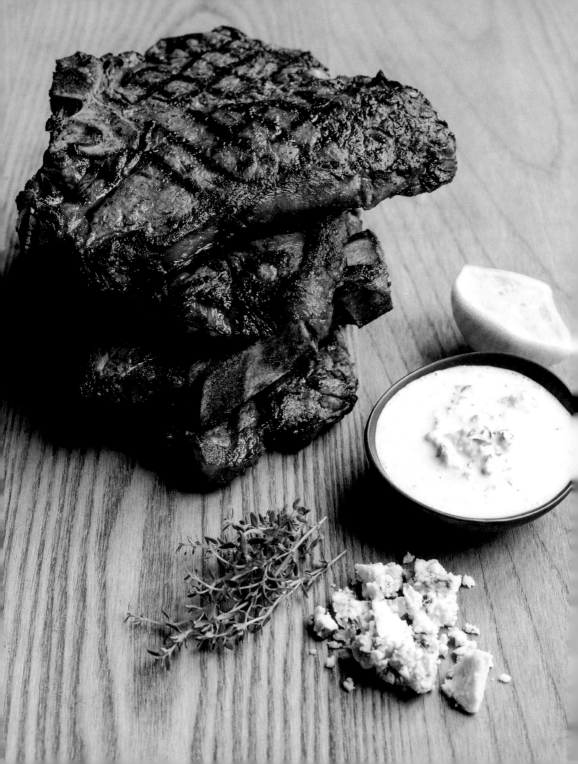

GRILLED T-BONES WITH BLUE CHEESE DRESSING & RADICCHIO SLAW

Some special occasions call for a stack of steaks. Coconut oil adds rich flavor to the meat in this recipe, and it's a healthy substitute for butter, which is typically used in steak houses. Top the steak with Radicchio Slaw (see next page) or serve with fresh arugula and Caviar Lentils (see p. 261) for an indulgent and memorable meal. **Serves 4**

4 T-bone steaks
  (about 4 pounds)
2 tablespoons coconut oil,
  melted and divided
1 teaspoon coarse salt
½ teaspoon pepper
sprinkle of coarse sugar

BLUE CHEESE DRESSING

2 sprigs fresh thyme,
  stems removed
zest from half a lemon
¼ teaspoon coarse salt
⅛ teaspoon black pepper
pinch of coarse sugar
¼ cup buttermilk
1 heaping tablespoon blue
  cheese, plus additional
  to taste
juice from half a lemon

Heat the grill. Let steaks warm to room temperature. Brush with coconut oil, then season both sides of the steaks generously with coarse salt, pepper, and a sprinkle of coarse sugar.

Place the steaks on the grill. The cooking time will depend on the thickness of the steak. A 1-inch steak will take 4–5 minutes on each side to cook to medium. (Just 1–2 minutes more will cook it to medium-well.) Continue to brush the meat with the leftover coconut oil while the steak is on the grill. Once the steaks are done, let them rest a few minutes before serving.

TO MAKE THE DRESSING: In a small bowl, mix together the thyme, lemon zest, salt, pepper, and sugar. Whisk in buttermilk and blue cheese. Finish with a burst of lemon juice and more blue cheese chunks, if desired.

Drizzle any remaining coconut oil over the steaks and top with dressing just before serving.

Radicchio Slaw

This is a fresh, tart slaw that pairs especially well with beef, pork, eggs, and other rich dishes. It's also tasty on an omelet. • The pickled green peppercorns are readily stocked at Italian or Mediterranean markets, but you can pick any salty pickled item that looks fun. **Serves 4**

1 small head radicchio, chopped
1 tablespoon thinly sliced
   shallot or red onion
¼ cup chopped fresh basil
¼ cup chopped fresh parsley
1 sprig fresh thyme, chopped
½ cup chopped green olives
½ 2-ounce tin anchovies in oil,
   chopped
1 teaspoon pickled green
   peppercorns or capers
2 tablespoons extra-virgin
   olive oil
juice from 2 lemons

Combine radicchio, shallot or onion, herbs, olives, and anchovies, plus the pickled peppercorns, if using, in a large bowl. Toss with olive oil and lemon juice to coat.

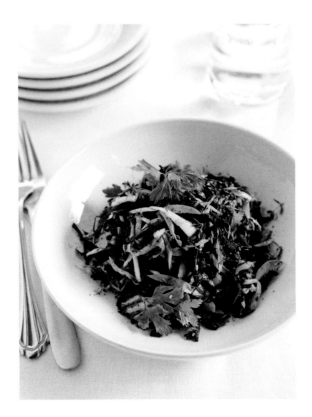

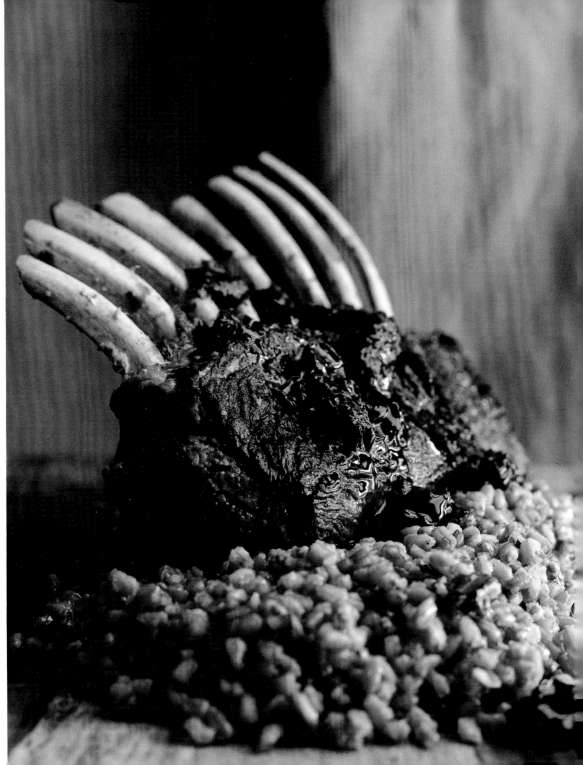

TECHNIQUE

FRESH SLAWS

I love to finish a dish with fresh-chopped slaw. Think of slaw as a small salad that is mixed in with your meal. Really, it's not so different from throwing some lettuce and fresh-cut tomatoes on top of a taco.

The possibilities are endless with slaws, which can be put together with a wide variety of crunchy vegetables. Cabbage makes an excellent base—it's crunchy, affordable, and good for your gut. Here are some guidelines to help you build your own finishing touch.

Start with a thinly sliced crunchy base:
cabbage, kale, fennel, kohlrabi, carrots, celery, bell peppers, crisp apples

There's no need for chopping here. I like to pull off the stems and use the whole leaf:
parsley, basil, cilantro

Toss with a squeeze of your favorite citrus:
lemon, lime, grapefruit, orange

Finish it off with seasoning to taste:
sprinkle of sugar, pinch of coarse salt, red pepper flakes or coarse ground pepper (optional)

Always use coarse salt to create another layer of texture.

Fennel Slaw

Fennel is in season from fall through early spring. It's commonly used in soups and stews, but I prefer to slice it up thin and serve it fresh. Delicately sweet in flavor, fennel is the perfect contrast to celery and caraway in this slaw, which also pairs well with fish. **Serves 6**

1 bulb fennel, thinly sliced into small strips
2 cups thinly sliced celery
½ cup coarsely chopped fresh flat-leaf parsley
2 teaspoons caraway seeds
2 tablespoons white wine vinegar
1 teaspoon coarse sugar
sprinkle of coarse pepper
juice from half a lemon

Combine the fennel, celery, parsley, and caraway seeds in a mixing bowl. Just before serving, add white wine vinegar, coarse sugar, pepper, and lemon juice and toss to coat. Adjust seasoning to taste.

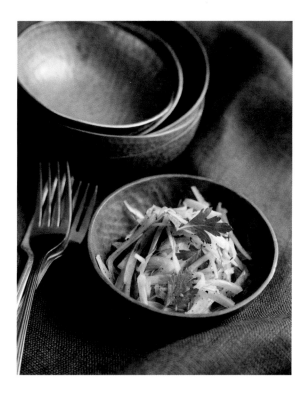

MORE TO SAVOR

If we were to avoid eating meat just one day a week,
this small change would have a big impact on both your
personal health and the health of our planet. If the cause
alone isn't compelling, these recipes will sell you on the idea.

MEATLESS

CHILLED SOBA WITH SPICY RED BEANS & POACHED EGGS

I like to enjoy this dish on a hot summer afternoon, however you could also serve it hot any time of the year. Many of these ingredients you'll already have on hand. **Serves 4**

2 teaspoons salt
4 eggs
1 15-ounce can red kidney beans or 2 cups cooked beans
½ pound bok choy or napa cabbage leaves, rolled lengthwise and thinly sliced (chiffonade)
2 cups carrots, cut into matchsticks
¼ cup thinly sliced red onion
2 tablespoons soy sauce, plus additional to taste
1 tablespoon chili paste (Sambal, p. 196), plus additional to taste
2 cups cooked and chilled soba noodles
4 cups hot or cold vegetable stock
drizzle of sesame oil
juice from 1 lemon

To poach the eggs, fill a shallow medium saucepan, halfway with water and add salt. Bring to a rolling boil and then crack the eggs into a small bowl one at a time and gently slide them into the boiling water. Cook for 5–6 minutes, or until the eggs are fully white. Drain with a slotted spoon and set aside.

If using canned beans, drain and rinse them. Combine the beans and vegetables in a mixing bowl. In a small bowl or measuring cup, stir together the soy sauce and chili paste. Pour the dressing over the beans and vegetables just before serving to keep them from wilting.

To assemble, divide the noodles into individual bowls. Sprinkle the dressed beans and vegetables on top of the noodles. Add one poached egg to each bowl. Pour in as much stock as you'd like, either cold or warm. To finish, drizzle with a small amount of sesame oil and a squeeze of lemon juice, adding additional soy sauce or chili paste to taste.

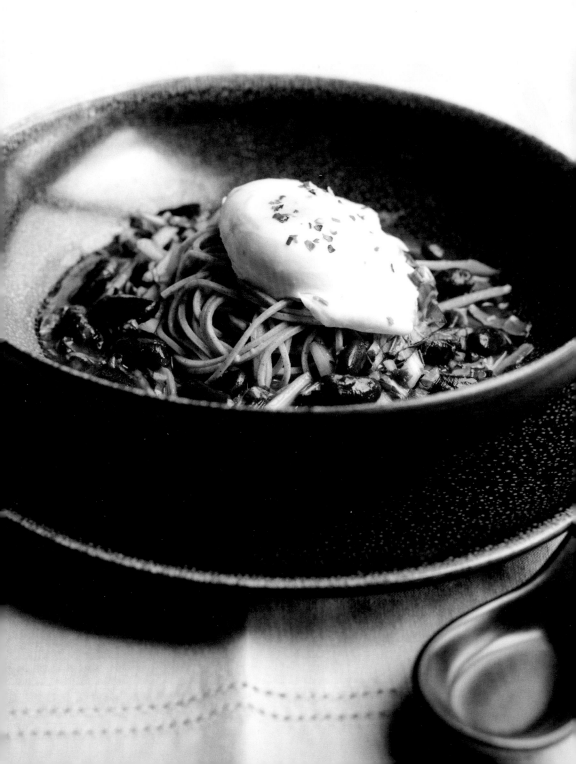

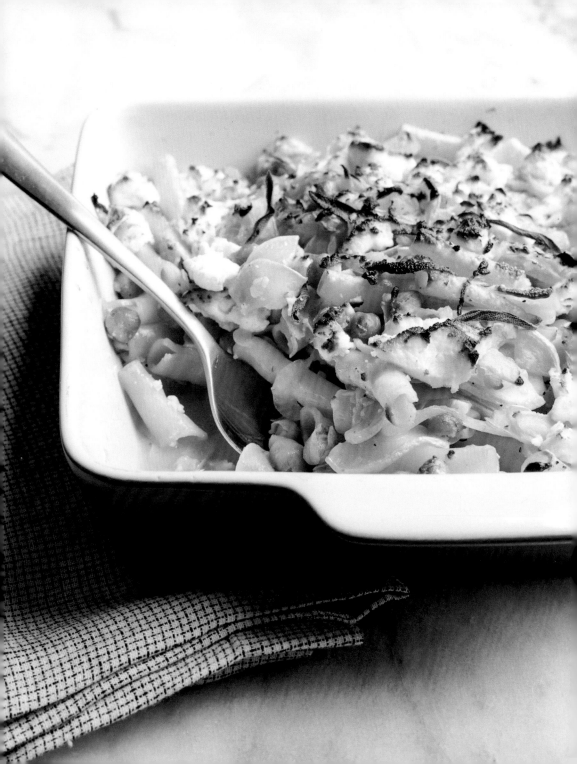

BAKED ZITI WITH TOASTED CHICKPEAS & SQUASH

This is a light dish that builds on the warmth of the toasted chickpeas. Slice the onion and squash really thin so you have delicate strips of color and flavor sitting in with the goat cheese and ziti. You can use any tube-shaped pasta, but more substantial noodles will hold up best in this baked dish. **Serves 4**

4 ounces uncooked ziti
2 tablespoons olive oil, divided
1 15-ounce can chickpeas or
    2 cups cooked chickpeas
¼ teaspoon coriander
1 pound yellow squash, sliced
    thin (about 3 cups)
1 cup thinly sliced white or
    yellow onion
1½ cups vegetable stock
coarse salt and pepper to taste
4 ounces goat cheese,
    crumbled
2 small sprigs of fresh sage,
    stems removed

Heat the oven to 400 degrees.

Bring a large pot of salted water to a boil and add the ziti. Cook until not quite al dente—the pasta will finish cooking in the oven. Remove from heat, drain the pasta, and set it aside.

While the pasta is cooking, warm 1 tablespoon of olive oil in a large pan over medium-high heat. If using canned chickpeas, drain and rinse them. Add the chickpeas and coriander and toast until golden brown, about 5–6 minutes, stirring to get even color.

Add the squash and onions to the chickpeas and sauté until they soften. Add the stock and cook for a couple minutes more, until the stock cooks down a bit and looks thick and bubbly. Season to taste with salt and pepper.

Remove from heat and gently fold in the cooked pasta, then transfer it all to a 9-inch square pan and top with crumbled goat cheese and sage. Bake on the middle rack of the oven for 10 minutes. Finish baking an additional 5–10 minutes on the top rack of the oven to get a nice golden brown color. Drizzle with the remaining 1 tablespoon of olive oil and serve hot.

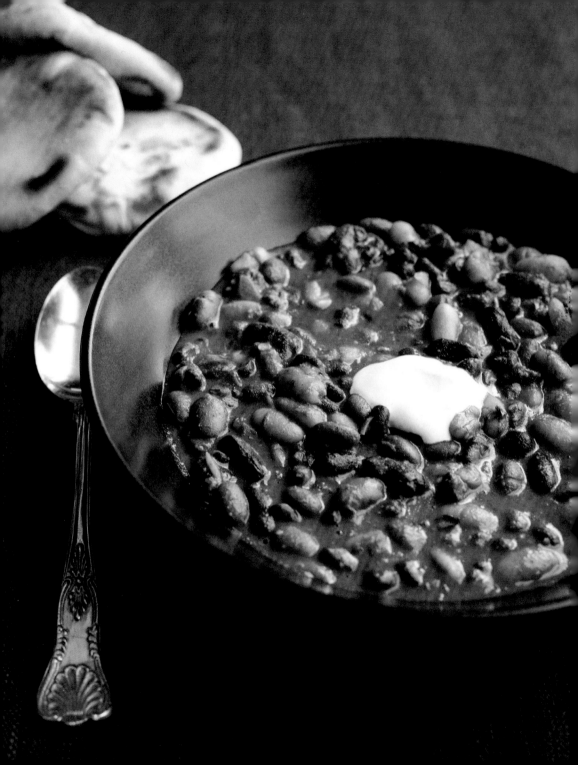

MIXED BEAN CURRY

It probably goes without saying that cooked beans will give this dish a superior texture and flavor . . . but don't let that keep you from enjoying this vegetarian curry dish. With canned beans you can be done in about 15 minutes! Any combination of beans will do—I like to use a little of everything. **Serves 6**

2 tablespoons coconut oil
1 tablespoon minced fresh
    ginger
1 tablespoon minced garlic
2 cups diced onions
¼ cup Madras curry powder
1 cup puréed or crushed
    tomatoes, canned or fresh
4 cups vegetable stock
1 13.5-ounce can coconut milk
¼ cup minced jalapeño
¼ cup chopped fresh cilantro
salt to taste
4 15-ounce cans beans (pinto
    beans, great northern beans,
    chickpeas, red kidney beans)
    or 6 cups cooked beans

ON TOP
¼ cup plain yogurt
1 jalapeño, sliced and sprinkled
    with salt

Warm the coconut oil in a large stockpot over medium-high heat. Add the ginger and garlic and sauté just a minute or two. Then add the onions and cook until they are golden brown on the edges.

Add the curry powder. Cook, continuously scraping the bottom of the pan, until fragrant. Add the tomatoes and stir until combined, then add stock and bring to low rolling boil.

Stir in the coconut milk until fully incorporated, then add the jalapeño and cilantro. Mix it all together and salt to taste. If using canned beans, drain and rinse them. Add the beans to the pot. Gently fold together without crushing the beans.

Serve as a hearty soup or over rice with a dollop of plain yogurt and jalapeño to taste.

COOKING DRY BEANS

This is a technique that requires little hands-on time, but it does take some planning.

1

Start by soaking the beans in cold water. For larger varieties, such as butter beans or large lima beans, you'll want to soak them for just a couple of hours. Other varieties will do well soaking overnight. Just to be safe, store the beans in the refrigerator—it's fine if it takes a full 24 hours to get back to them.

2

Once the beans have about doubled in size, drain them and rinse thoroughly. Pour the beans into a large pot and fill with fresh water. Stir in a teaspoon of salt and bring the pot to a rolling boil over high heat, then reduce heat to low and let simmer for at least 1 hour. The beans will be soft yet still have a bite when adequately cooked. Remove from heat and set aside to cool for 5–10 minutes before draining the water. This will keep the beans from shriveling up.

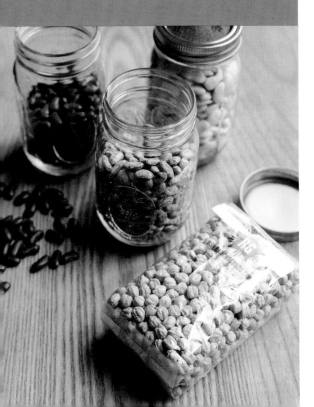

Caviar Lentils

This lentil variety cooks up as tiny little black pearls that look just like caviar, hence the name. Toss them in a bit of olive oil with some salt and your favorite seasonings and scoop onto toasted bread or scrambled eggs. **Serves 6**

3 cups water or vegetable stock
1 cup black caviar lentils
1 teaspoon coarse salt
1 tablespoon extra-virgin olive oil
juice from half a lemon
salt and pepper to taste

Rinse and sort the lentils to remove any debris or discolored lentils.

In a small stockpot, bring the water or stock to a boil over high heat. Add lentils and 1 teaspoon salt. Return to a low rolling boil, then reduce heat and cook for about 15 minutes, or until the lentils are tender and most of the moisture has been absorbed. Remove from heat, cover, and let rest a minute.

Drain out any excess liquid, then drizzle with olive oil, lemon juice, and salt and pepper to taste.

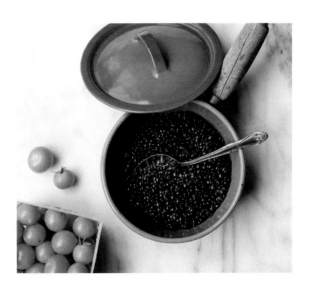

FALAFEL WITH CHUNKY CUCUMBER YOGURT SAUCE

By now you know I'm a big fan of chickpeas—so it's time to pay homage to the chickpea "meatball." Falafel is a delightful vegetarian protein that you can enjoy with or without a pita. If you go the traditional route, stack up your pita with fresh greens, Chunky Cucumber Yogurt Sauce, and falafel. Alternatively, falafel balls sit pretty atop a Greek salad. For a full-on Mediterranean experience, serve up the Classic Hummus (see p. 91) as a starter. **Serves 4**

1 15-ounce can chickpeas or
   2 cups cooked chickpeas
up to ¼ cup chickpea flour
1 egg
1 tablespoon minced parsley
1 teaspoon minced garlic
1 teaspoon cumin
1 teaspoon coriander
½ teaspoon paprika
¼ cup olive oil
4 medium-sized pitas
4 cups loose-leaf greens

CHUNKY CUCUMBER YOGURT SAUCE

1 cup plain Greek yogurt
1 tablespoon chopped fresh dill
½ cup cucumber, chopped
4 pickled pepperoncini,
   chopped small
2 tablespoons chopped fresh
   chives
1 tablespoon minced red onion
1 tablespoon extra-virgin
   olive oil
juice from half a lemon
¼ teaspoon salt

TO MAKE THE CUCUMBER YOGURT: Combine the ingredients in a small bowl and fold together. Chill until ready to serve.

TO MAKE THE FALAFEL: Pulse the chickpeas in a food processor until you have a thick, crumbly paste. Add 2 tablespoons of chickpea flour to the chickpea paste along with the egg, parsley, garlic, and spices. Pulse to combine. If the mixture is not holding together, add more flour, 1 tablespoon at a time. Shape the chickpea mixture into 12 falafel, each about the size of a golf ball.

Heat the olive oil in a sauté pan over medium heat. Place half of the falafel in the pan. Gently sauté, turning with tongs to get an even golden brown color and crisp exterior, about 6–8 minutes per batch.

While you are finishing up the falafel, warm the pitas in a dry pan over medium heat to make them more pliable.

Pile each pita with greens, cucumber yogurt, and 3 falafel and serve.

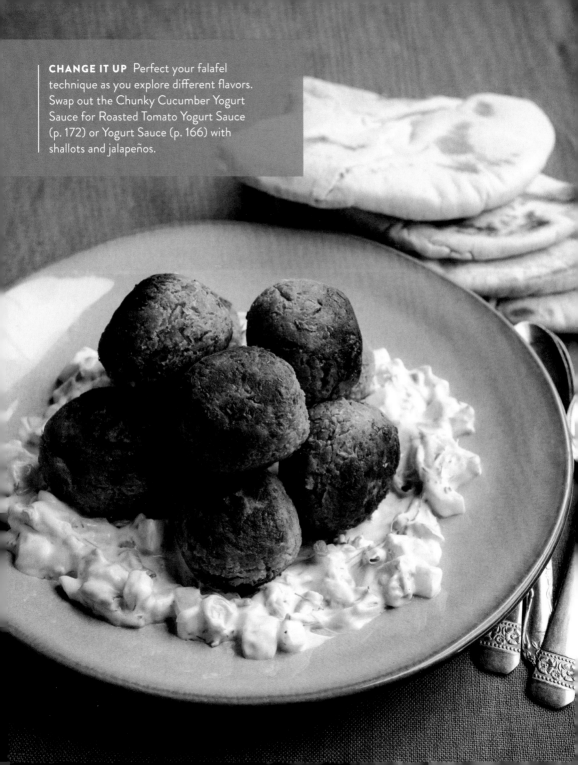

CHANGE IT UP Perfect your falafel technique as you explore different flavors. Swap out the Chunky Cucumber Yogurt Sauce for Roasted Tomato Yogurt Sauce (p. 172) or Yogurt Sauce (p. 166) with shallots and jalapeños.

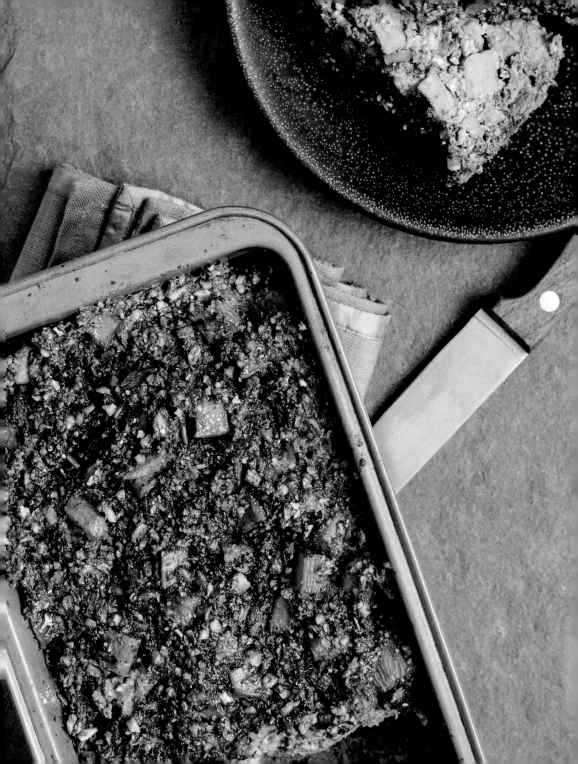

SWEET POTATO, PECAN & MUSHROOM "MEATLOAF"

This pecan and mushroom "meatloaf" has a hearty texture and enough flavor to stand in for steak with no apologies. Serve it up just like a traditional meatloaf, with a heaping spoonful of your favorite barbecue sauce or gravy, alongside buttered potatoes or simple noodles. Slice up any leftovers for sandwiches or crumble into burritos or tacos. We used Italian seasoning, and the flavor was terrific. Feel free to substitute your favorite seasoning in its place. **Serves 8**

4 cups peeled and cubed sweet potatoes
1 pound mushrooms
2 cups pecan pieces
2 cups cubed gluten-free bread, lightly packed
3 eggs, lightly beaten
4 teaspoons Italian seasoning
2 tablespoons gluten-free flour
½ teaspoon coarse salt (increase to 1 teaspoon if your seasoning blend doesn't include salt)
1 teaspoon coarsely ground pepper

Heat the oven to 350 degrees. Lightly grease a standard loaf pan with nonstick cooking spray or coconut oil.

Boil the sweet potatoes in water until fork tender, approximately 8 minutes. Drain thoroughly and set aside. They will be slightly undercooked.

In a food processor, combine the mushrooms, pecans, and bread, and pulse until the mixture is crumbly. Transfer to a large mixing bowl. Add the eggs, seasoning, gluten-free flour, salt, and pepper and stir until well combined. Gently fold in the cooked sweet potatoes.

Transfer the mixture to the prepared loaf pan. Place on the middle rack of the oven and bake for about 1 hour, or until the center of the loaf feels firm to the touch.

Note: Regular bread and all-purpose flour can be substituted for the gluten-free ingredients specified.

DELICIOUS WITH GRILLED ROMAINE (P. 123), WITH OR WITHOUT THE PANCETTA.

EGGPLANT & ONION
FRIED WILD RICE

Fried rice is a great meal to have in your repertoire. There are countless variations in every culture. Dishes like this one can be reinvented from week to week to feature whatever great finds turn up at the farmers' market or to sub in leftovers (bacon or meat, or even the rice). Serve fried rice as a side or as the main event—thanks to the eggs and vegetables, it's a balanced meal for a busy night. **Serves 4**

2 cups wild rice
3 cups water (more if
   specified on package)
olive oil
3 cups diced eggplant
1 cup minced white onion
1 tablespoon minced garlic
4 eggs, lightly beaten
½ teaspoon coarse salt
1 teaspoon sesame oil
freshly grated Parmesan

Start the rice and water in the rice cooker. If you don't have a rice cooker, bring a pot of salted water to a rolling boil and add the rice. Cover and reduce heat to low. Let simmer as directed on the package. Most wild rice varieties require 40–45 minutes to cook.

When the rice is about 20 minutes from being finished, prepare the other ingredients. Coat the bottom of a large nonstick sauté pan with olive oil and bring to medium-high heat. Add the diced eggplant, onion, and garlic and panfry it until it becomes golden brown. The eggplant will soak up the olive oil, so add more if needed.

Add the eggs to the eggplant mixture, and scramble until firm. When the rice is finished cooking, add it to the eggplant mixture along with the salt, stirring until thoroughly combined. Remove from heat. Drizzle with sesame oil and sprinkle with Parmesan before serving.

Note: To use leftover white or brown rice in this dish, get a pot ready and add a splash of water to 3 cups cooked rice. Warm over medium heat with the lid on for 8–10 minutes, stirring periodically. The extra water will keep the rice from drying out and will help it cook up more evenly in the finished dish.

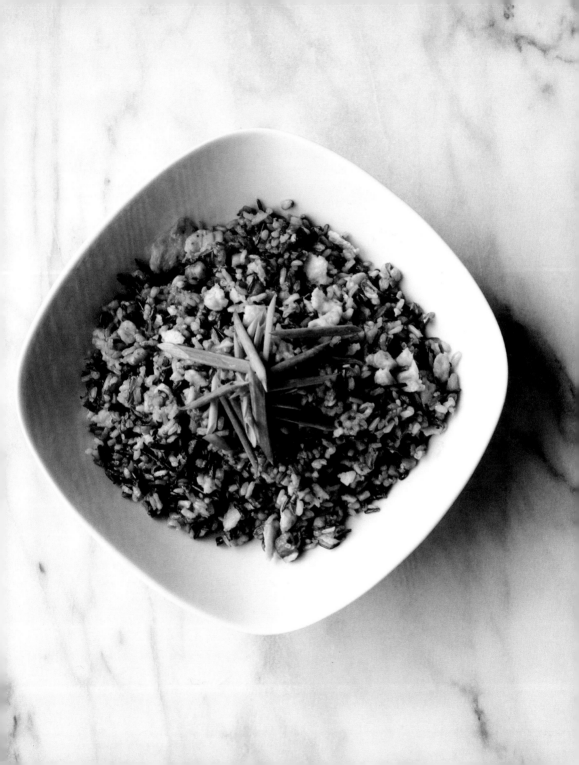

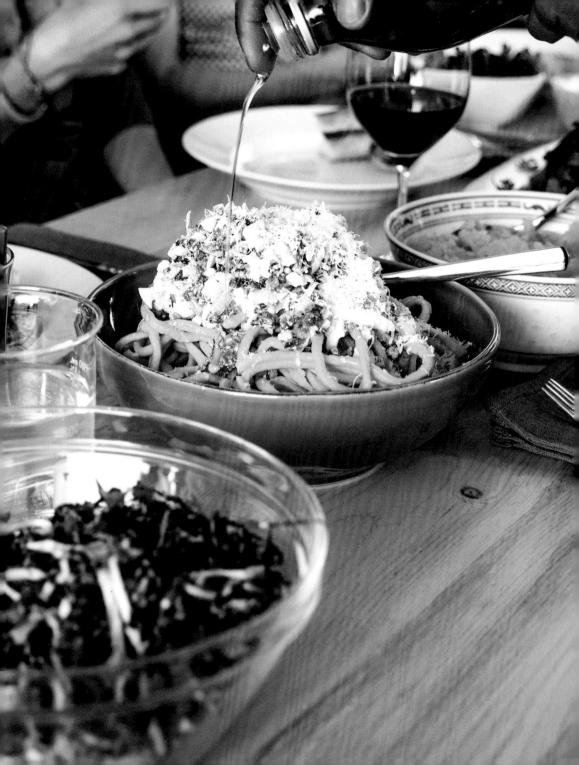

HOMEMADE EGG PASTA WITH FRESH-CHOPPED SAUCE

Pasta doesn't have to be topped with a bubbling hot sauce to taste good. The briny flavor of this sauce is especially delicious with homemade egg pasta. Serve the pasta while it's still warm with plenty of high-quality Parmesan on top—it's one of the ingredients you don't want to skimp on. **Serves 4**

2 cups all-purpose flour
4 eggs, lightly beaten

FRESH-CHOPPED SAUCE

2 hard-boiled eggs, chopped
½ 2-ounce tin anchovies in oil, chopped (optional)
½ cup chopped fresh parsley
2 cloves minced garlic
1 tablespoon capers, drained
juice from 1 lemon
2 tablespoons extra-virgin olive oil
salt and pepper to taste

ON TOP

freshly grated Parmesan
extra-virgin olive oil

Pile the flour on a flat work surface or into a flat-bottomed bowl and make a well in the center. Pour in the eggs. Using a fork, mix the eggs into the flour little by little. The dough should be elastic but not sticky. If it's too dry and not holding together, add in a splash of water. If it's too sticky, add a bit more flour. Once the mixture is thoroughly incorporated, set it aside to rest for about 30 minutes. Skip this step and your pasta probably won't hold up.

Roll out the pasta into thin, oblong sheets either by running it through a pasta maker or simply using a rolling pin. Dust with flour frequently to keep the dough from sticking.

To cut your pasta, roll up the flat sheet of dough tightly, starting from the shorter side. Use a sharp knife to cut it into strips as wide as you would like. Cook in a large pot of salted water at a low rolling boil. Fresh pasta will float when it's fully cooked.

TO MAKE THE SAUCE: Combine all the ingredients in a small bowl. Pile on top of the homemade pasta and finish with freshly grated Parmesan and a drizzle of extra-virgin olive oil.

SEE THE HOMEMADE PASTA TECHNIQUE ON PAGE 152.

LITTLE BIT

We love dessert for the way it makes us feel.
These recipes often use honey in place of refined sugar
and coconut oil rather than butter.
Don't forget that our drinks can also double as dessert.

SWEET

BANANA MOUSSE DESSERT

This is an easy, guilt-free dessert that you can make in advance. By alternating layers of banana mousse and yogurt, you get a taste of sweet, creamy, and toasted nut flavors in a single spoonful. No one has to know how easy it was to make. **Serves 4**

4 ripe bananas (reserve half
    a banana for garnish)
1 tablespoon light molasses
1 tablespoon honey or
    maple syrup
¼ teaspoon cinnamon
¼ teaspoon vanilla or
    almond extract
½ cup peanuts or walnuts
1 cup plain Greek yogurt

Place the bananas in a food processor with the molasses, honey or maple syrup, cinnamon, and vanilla or almond extract. Pulse until smooth.

In a dry pan over medium-high heat, toast the nuts until they become fragrant and golden brown. Remove from heat and set aside to cool.

Spoon the banana mousse mixture into individual bowls. Top with a generous dollop of yogurt and then sprinkle with toasted peanuts or walnuts. Add a bit more banana mousse and garnish with sliced banana and another dusting of toasted nuts.

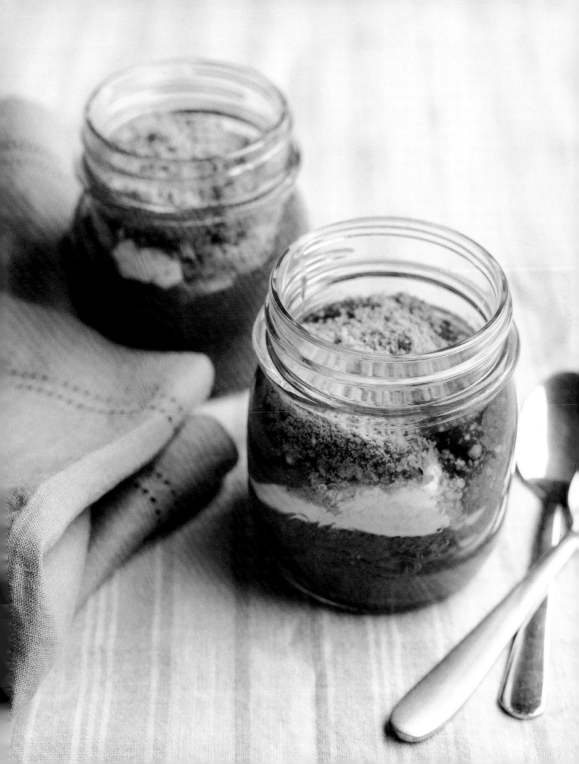

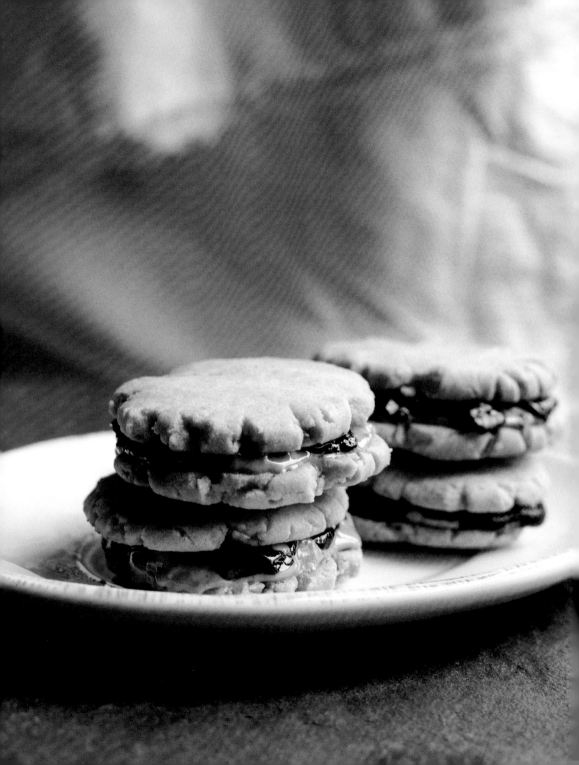

PB&J COOKIES

Here the idea was to re-create a favorite snack from my childhood—actually it continues to be a favorite of mine. Who says peanut butter and jelly can't come together in a pretty dessert? It might seem a bit fussy to make sandwich cookies at home, but the end result is both nostalgic and delicious. **Serves 10**

1 cup coconut oil
1 egg
1 cup refined sugar
1 teaspoon vanilla extract
2 cups all-purpose flour
½ teaspoon baking powder
½ teaspoon baking soda
¼ teaspoon salt

PB&J FILLING
½ cup natural peanut butter
¼ cup grape jelly or fruit
  preserves

Heat the oven to 350 degrees. Line a large baking sheet with parchment paper.

In a mixing bowl, combine the coconut oil, egg, sugar, and vanilla and stir with a wooden spoon until well combined. Add in the dry ingredients and work the dough until it holds together. It may seem crumbly at first, but keep working it (don't be afraid to use your hands).

Portion out 20 small balls, each about the size of a golf ball, and place them onto the baking sheet. Gently flatten each ball before placing the cookies in the oven.

Bake cookies for 12–15 minutes. While they are still slightly warm, spread half of the cookies with peanut butter and jelly, and top with a second cookie. Serve with milk. Makes 10 sandwich cookies.

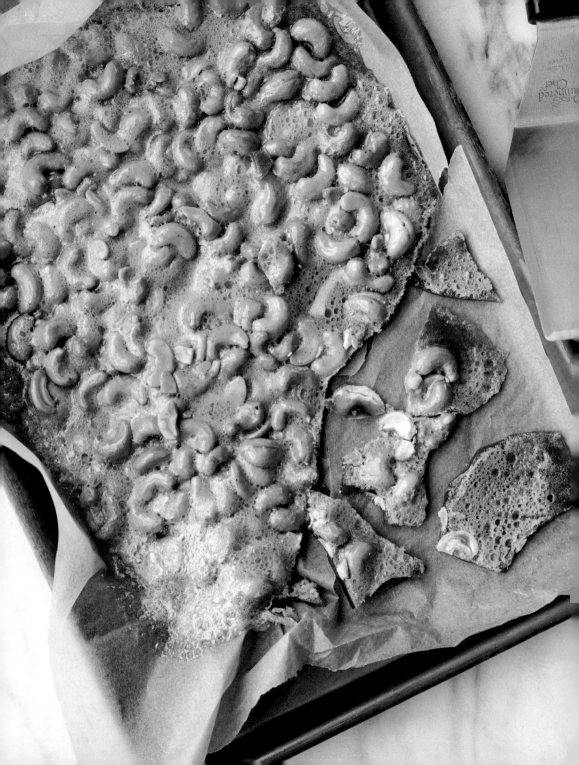

CASHEW HONEY BRITTLE

There is a magical tipping point when sweets caramelize and turn into candy. To pull it off you need a candy thermometer and an oven mitt to keep from burning your hands. The best news of all is that you don't have to use corn syrup to enjoy a little nut brittle! **Serves 8**

1 cup honey
¼ cup water
1 tablespoon butter
½ teaspoon vanilla extract
¼ teaspoon cinnamon
1 teaspoon baking soda
2 cups roasted and salted
   cashews

Line a small baking sheet with parchment paper.

In a heavy pot, combine the honey, water, butter, vanilla, and cinnamon and bring to a low rolling boil over medium-high heat, stirring constantly to keep the mixture from burning.

When the mixture begins to thicken and the color darkens, insert a candy thermometer and continue to cook until the temperature reaches 300 degrees.

Immediately remove the mixture from the heat and stir in baking soda and salted cashews. (The baking soda causes the brittle to expand, making it a bit more light and airy.)

Pour out the hot mixture onto the prepared baking sheet and set aside. As it cools, the honey mixture will harden. To speed up the process you can place the baking sheet in the freezer.

Serve with a scoop of ice cream or frozen yogurt or as a stand-alone treat.

BAKED GRANOLA CRISP

This simple dessert tastes like baked oatmeal, a treat that I don't like to relegate to breakfast. Simply prepare the homemade granola in advance or use granola that you have on hand. You can use other fruit instead of bananas—apples or blueberries also taste great. **Serves 6**

3 cups granola, homemade
   or packaged
2 cups almond milk
1 banana, coarsely chopped
sprinkle of cinnamon
   or nutmeg
maple syrup to finish

HOMEMADE GRANOLA

2 cups old-fashioned rolled
   oats
½ cup brown sugar
½ cup unsweetened dried
   shredded coconut
½ cup maple syrup or agave
2 tablespoons unfiltered
   apple juice
2 tablespoons coconut oil,
   melted
¼ cup dried fruit or nuts
   (optional)

TO MAKE THE GRANOLA: Heat the oven to 300 degrees. Line a large baking sheet with parchment paper or foil.

In a large bowl, combine oats, brown sugar, and shredded coconut, and stir to combine. Then add the maple syrup or agave, apple juice, and coconut oil. Stir until the oat mixture is evenly distributed. Add another splash of apple juice if the granola seems too dry. Let the granola mixture sit for about 10 minutes before baking to fully absorb the liquid.

Bake for 45 minutes, then add the dried fruit or nuts, if desired, and bake for an additional 10–15 minutes, or until the granola is golden brown. Makes about 3 cups.

TO MAKE THE CRISP: Increase the oven temperature to 350 degrees.

Place 3 cups of granola in a mixing bowl and add the milk and banana. Stir until well combined. Spoon into individual ramekins or oven-safe cups and sprinkle with cinnamon or nutmeg.

Bake for 20 minutes. Drizzle with maple syrup just before serving.

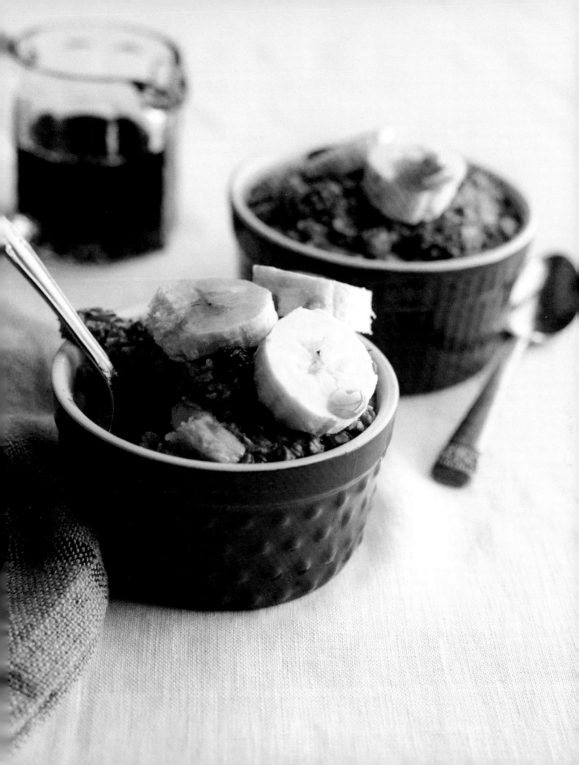

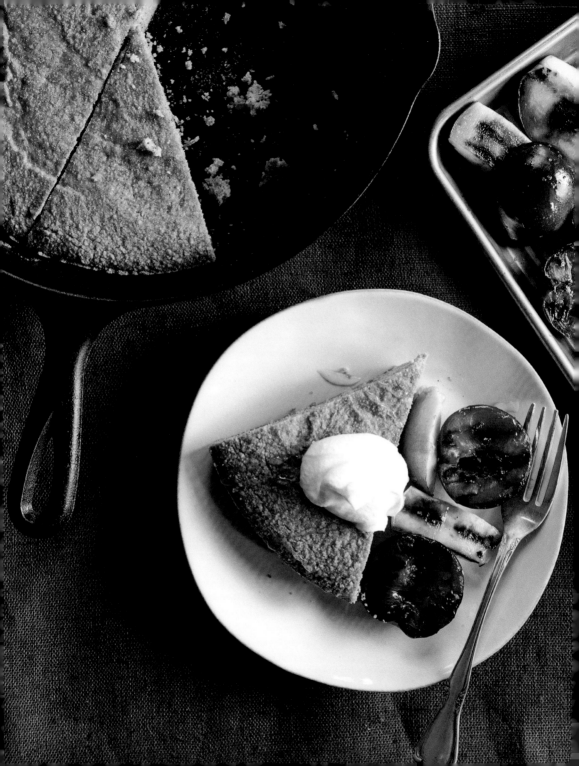

ALMOND CORNBREAD
WITH GRILLED STONE FRUIT

This is a delicious gluten-free cornbread that you can serve as a great dessert or hearty side to your meal. Dense with healthy fats and protein, almond meal is a fantastic gluten-free flour that is easy to work with and yields a rich, moist cornbread or cake that doesn't feel heavy. • Corn flour will give you a smoother texture than cornmeal. **Serves 8**

2 cups almond meal
2 cups fine-ground cornmeal
4 eggs
2 cups milk
½ cup sugar
2 teaspoons ground cinnamon
1 teaspoon baking soda
½ teaspoon salt

GRILLED STONE FRUIT

8 pieces stone fruit (peaches, apricots, or nectarines)
olive oil
sprinkle of coarse sugar

ON TOP

plain Greek yogurt
honey
cinnamon

Heat the oven to 350 degrees. Blend all the ingredients together in a large bowl until thoroughly combined. The mixture will be thick and smooth. Let rest for 30 minutes if you have the time.

Pour the cornbread batter into a lightly greased 10-inch cast-iron skillet (a 9 × 13–inch baking dish also works) and bake for 60 minutes, or until the center is set.

With about 10 minutes to go on the cornbread, heat the grill to high. Cut the fruit in half, remove the pit, and brush the flesh with olive oil. Add a sprinkle of sugar. Grill the fruit cut-side down for 3–5 minutes or just long enough to warm the fruit and make some lovely grill marks.

Serve up the grilled stone fruit alongside your almond cornbread. With a spoonful of Greek yogurt, a drizzle of honey, and a hit of cinnamon, this makes a fantastic dessert.

DARK CHOCOLATE BARK WITH SPICED PUMPKIN SEEDS

I couldn't resist another brittle, and this one is low maintenance for sure. Why pay for store-bought bark when you can make it in under 20 minutes at home? Cayenne pepper and pumpkin seeds make this simple dessert unique. I like to finish it off with a good sprinkle of Maldon salt—it adds a bit more flavor and texture—but coarse salt works just fine too. **Serves 8**

2 cups dark chocolate chips
½ cup (1 stick) butter
1 cup pepitas (shelled,
   unsalted pumpkin seeds)
1 teaspoon cayenne pepper,
   plus more for finishing
1 teaspoon Maldon salt or
   coarse salt

Line a 9 × 13–inch baking sheet with parchment paper.

In a dry pan over medium-high heat, toast the pumpkin seeds for about 5 minutes or until they become fragrant.

Melt the chocolate chips and butter in a water bath by placing them in a metal bowl on top of a pot of boiling water and stirring until the mixture is smooth and fully melted. Remove from heat and stir in the pumpkin seeds and cayenne pepper.

Pour the chocolate mixture onto the prepared baking sheet and tip the pan to evenly distribute. Top with salt and another sprinkle of cayenne pepper.

Place the baking sheet in the freezer for 20 minutes to set. Keep cool until you are ready to serve, then break apart into pieces.

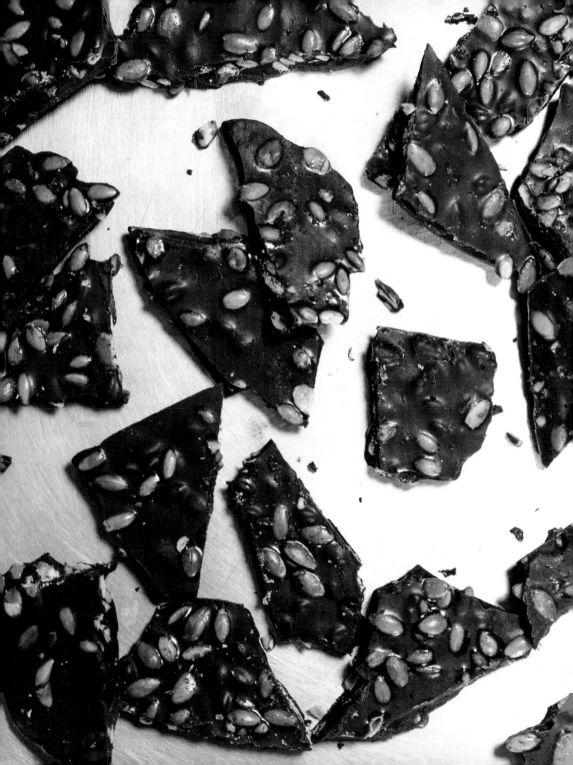

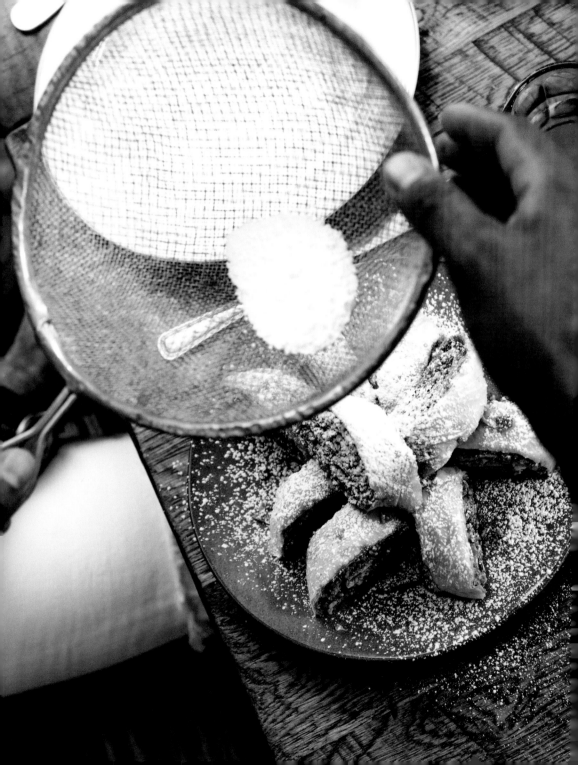

BAKLAVA

This classic Middle Eastern dessert goes well with most anything. Look for a high-quality phyllo to simplify the process. You can store the unused dough in the freezer for another occasion, since a 1-pound box makes three batches of baklava. **Serves 10**

1 cup cashews or shelled
   green pistachios
1 cup walnut pieces
½ cup whole currants
   or chopped raisins
½ cup brown sugar
1 tablespoon cinnamon
6 sheets of phyllo dough
1 cup coconut oil or butter,
   melted

ON TOP
¼ cup powdered sugar
2 tablespoons maple syrup
   or honey

Heat the oven to 375 degrees.

Combine the nuts, dried fruit, brown sugar, and cinnamon in a food processor and pulse a few times until you have a thick, chunky mixture. Set aside.

Working with the pastry dough is the only part that is slightly tricky. The key is to gently brush each sheet with melted coconut oil or butter. Place a long sheet of parchment paper on a clean work surface and lay down a single sheet of phyllo. After you have brushed it thoroughly with oil or butter, lay another sheet directly on top and repeat the process until you have a stack of 6 sheets.

Spread the nut mixture evenly across the stack of phyllo pastry. The dough can tear easily, so use a light touch.

Starting from one of the longer sides, begin rolling the dough away from you, being careful to keep the roll tight.

Finally, use a sharp knife to cut the roll into thick pinwheels. Use the parchment paper to transfer the roll to a large baking sheet.

Bake on the top rack of the oven for 10 minutes, then rotate the pan and bake for 5 more minutes, or until pastry is golden brown.

Dust with powdered sugar and drizzle with maple syrup or honey before serving.

Note: If you find you have leftover filling, keep it in a jar and add a spoonful or three to your morning oatmeal.

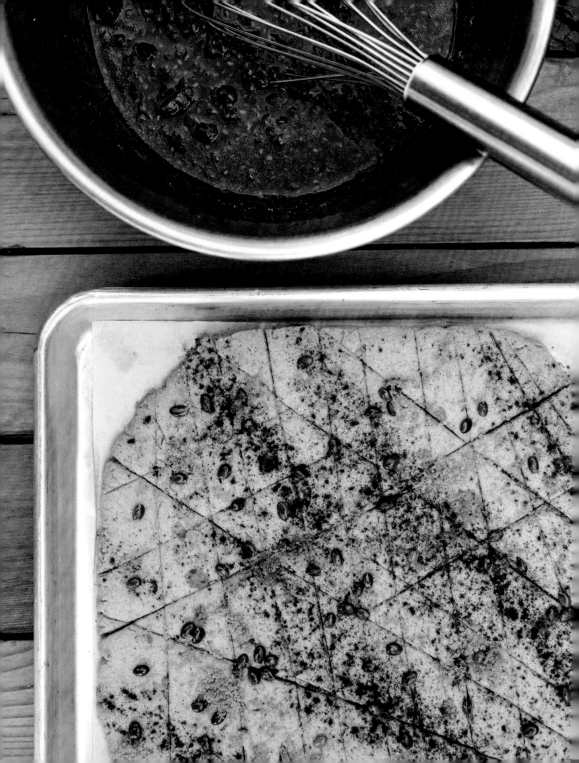

CINNAMON SHORTBREAD COOKIES WITH FRESH JAM

Back in the day at Alameda High School we did an epic ride from Denver to Taos, New Mexico. As soon as we got off the bike, we were greeted with warm fresh-baked biscochitos, a shortbread cookie commonly served in the Southwest. Many recipes call for lard, so I've come up with my own interpretation here in hopes of encouraging you to try these cookies for yourself. Serve with bowls of smashed berries and honey—my take on fresh jam. **Serves 10**

1 tablespoon anise seeds
   or fennel seeds
1 tablespoon vanilla extract
¾ cup packed brown sugar
¾ cup coconut oil or butter,
   softened
2 eggs
splash of brandy (optional)
3 cups all-purpose flour
1 teaspoon baking powder
1 tablespoon cinnamon,
   plus additional on top
¼ teaspoon salt

FRESH JAM
1 pint fresh raspberries
¼ cup honey

Heat the oven to 350 degrees. Line a baking sheet with parchment paper.

Soak the anise or fennel seeds in the vanilla while you prepare the dough.

In a mixing bowl, combine brown sugar, coconut oil or butter, eggs, and brandy, if using. Stir the mixture together until the sugar is fully incorporated.

In a separate bowl, combine the flour, baking powder, cinnamon, and salt.

Strain the vanilla and add it to the wet ingredients, reserving the anise or fennel. Then combine the wet and dry ingredients and knead the dough until it holds together and the texture becomes smooth and even. Shape the dough into a ball and place it on the prepared baking sheet.

Use a rolling pin or wine bottle to roll it out until it's about ¼-inch thick. Scatter the anise seeds or fennel on top of the dough and lightly press them in with the palm of your hand. Score the dough with a sharp knife so it will easily break apart into bite-sized servings— I like making uneven cuts to form geometric shapes. (You can also use cookie cutters.)

(recipe continues)

Sprinkle with more cinnamon and bake the cookies on the middle rack of the oven for 15–20 minutes, or until they are no longer soft to the touch. Remove from oven to cool completely before breaking the cookies apart.

TO MAKE THE FRESH JAM: While the cookies are baking, combine the raspberries and honey in a small mixing bowl and mash with a wire whisk. The mixture will be thinner than traditional jam. Serve the fresh jam alongside the cookies for dipping.

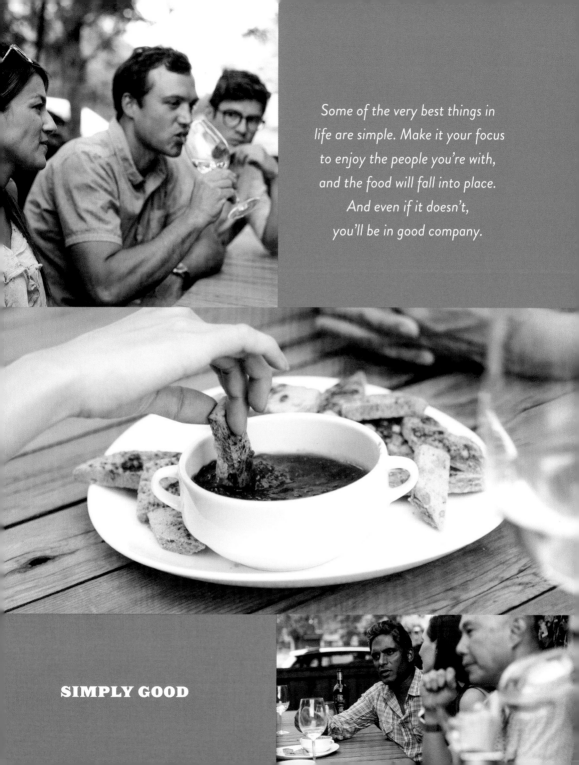

Some of the very best things in
life are simple. Make it your focus
to enjoy the people you're with,
and the food will fall into place.
And even if it doesn't,
you'll be in good company.

SIMPLY GOOD

SHIFT GEARS

*While we often worry about what we need to eat
to perform better, how we eat and who we eat with
matter more than what we eat. Be intentional
about cooking and sharing meals with others.*

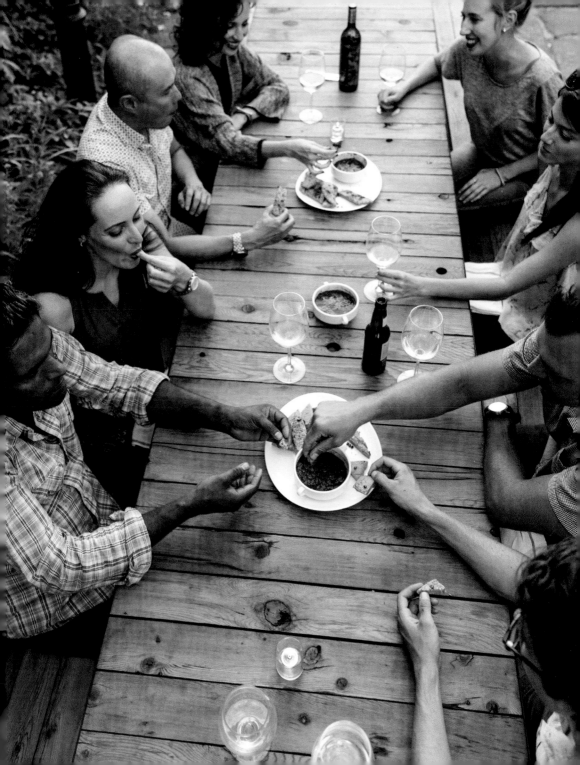

NUTRITION FACTS

Carbohydrates, protein, and fat have become political parties. They all work. You can use the stats that follow to find the agenda that best fits your biology. Keep in mind that the recipes are just suggestions—change it up as needed.

DRINKS

	SERVINGS	CALORIES	PROTEIN (G)	CARBS (G)	FAT (G)	FIBER (G)	SODIUM (MG)
Homemade Hot Chocolate	4	263	3	30	18	4	114
Lemon Hibiscus Iced Tea with Honey	6	28	---	7	---	---	6
Mumbai Spiced Chai	6	70	4	11	1	---	59
Salty Cucumber Lime Soda	6	25	---	7	---	---	813
Sparkling Ginger Soda	6	83	---	21	---	1	52
Spiced Apple Cider (with Rim Topper)	6	135	---	33	---	---	25
Swiss Mountain Herb Tea	6	36	---	11	---	1	4
Vietnamese-Style Coffee	4	135	6	13	7	---	92
Watermelon Soda with Fresh Mint	6	31	1	8	---	---	51

STARTERS

	SERVINGS	CALORIES	PROTEIN (G)	CARBS (G)	FAT (G)	FIBER (G)	SODIUM (MG)
Bitter Chard on Grilled Bread	6	383	8	41	22	3	483
Classic Hummus	4	209	6	16	14	5	663
Grilled Bread & Artichokes	8	245	10	45	4	5	641
Dipping Oil (1 tbsp. per serving)	8	125	---	1	14	---	1
Guacamole with Beans	8	153	3	13	11	6	175
Italian Rice Balls	8	426	11	50	20	2	414
Red Pepper Oil	8	35	---	1	4	---	74
Lemon Pesto	16	92	1	1	10	---	42
Toasted Chickpeas with Ghost Pepper Salt	4	124	5	15	---	5	687
Ghost Pepper Salt	18	3	---	1	---	---	1,565

STARTERS (continued)	SERVINGS	CALORIES	PROTEIN (G)	CARBS (G)	FAT (G)	FIBER (G)	SODIUM (MG)
Tuna Mushroom Salad with Lemon Tarragon Dressing	8	102	14	3	3	---	390
White Anchovy Toast	8	240	10	30	9	2	887

SIDES SALADS SOUPS

	SERVINGS	CALORIES	PROTEIN (G)	CARBS (G)	FAT (G)	FIBER (G)	SODIUM (MG)
Beef Bone Stock* (1 cup per serving)	24	26	2	2	1	---	351
Broccoli Soup with Smoked Trout & Chives	6	101	8	15	2	4	1,052
Cauliflower & Corn Chowder with Red Pepper Oil	6	138	8	14	6	3	523
Chile & Lime–Spiced Bay Scallops	6	91	10	7	3	---	304
Chilled Black Bean Yogurt Soup	6	228	12	23	10	4	772
Citrus Salad with Yuzu Dressing & Wonton Crisps	6	201	3	16	15	2	145
Coconut Rice Porridge with Adacherri	4	239	3	31	10	1	637
Fresh Grapefruit & Avocado Salad	6	223	3	17	18	5	106
Grilled Romaine with Pancetta, Hard-Boiled Eggs	6	266	12	9	21	1	464
Dijon Dressing (1 tbsp. per serving)	6	83	---	---	9	---	158
Kimchee Spiced Salad (with Red Pepper Sesame Oil Dressing)	4	175	3	10	15	4	604
Olive Oil–Poached Tomato Soup with Walnuts	4	325	4	13	30	4	448
Pan-Roasted Chickpeas & Summer Vegetables	6	124	5	14	6	4	587
Pasta with Maple Carrots & Leeks	4	479	12	64	20	5	312
Spicy Red Beans & Rice	6	699	21	70	37	6	1,833
Sweet Potato–Stuffed Wonton Soup	6	359	12	47	14	4	1,647
Torn Bread & Radicchio Salad	6	274	7	26	17	3	376
Turkey Meatball & Tomato Soup	4	484	33	43	21	1	1,581
Vegetable Stock* (1 cup per serving)	16	3	---	---	---	---	2
Warm German Potato Salad	4	224	3	21	14	3	572

* **Note:** It is difficult to calculate nutritional information for stock because it is hard to say how much of the macronutrients actually end up in the stock.

CHICKEN

	SERVINGS	CALORIES	PROTEIN (G)	CARBS (G)	FAT (G)	FIBER (G)	SODIUM (MG)
Baked Chicken Parmesan	4	509	52	30	19	1	476
Bright & Chunky Marinara (¾ cup per serving)	8	93	3	14	4	4	264
Fresh Spinach Pasta	8	228	9	41	3	2	189
Chicken & Almond Dumplings	6	492	38	18	31	6	973
Chicken Madras	6	524	37	7	38	2	532
Harissa (2 tbsp. per serving)	12	87	2	9	6	4	202
Yogurt Sauce (2 tbsp. per serving)	6	33	2	3	1	---	75
Chicken Pad Thai	4	725	59	59	28	5	1,082
Chopped Chicken Salad	4	281	25	28	9	6	547
Pickled Onions & Radishes	4	11	---	2	---	---	296
Grilled Chicken with Homemade Barbecue Sauce	4	441	28	8	33	1	879
Kalamata Chicken with New Potatoes	6	406	31	38	14	5	1,067
Masala Chicken Wrap	6	279	23	30	8	1	551
Cabbage Slaw	6	12	---	3	---	1	103
Red Chicken	8	149	22	4	5	1	630
Baked Biriyani	8	278	6	60	2	3	321
Roasted Tomato Yogurt Sauce	12	44	2	4	3	---	126
Rustic Lemon Chicken	6	281	21	3	21	1	379
Sautéed Tortellini & Sausage with Collard Greens	6	508	21	39	30	3	884
Split Chicken with Lemon Garlic Sauce & Roasted Vegetables	6	606	43	18	41	6	684

SEAFOOD

	SERVINGS	CALORIES	PROTEIN (G)	CARBS (G)	FAT (G)	FIBER (G)	SODIUM (MG)
Baked Jambalaya	6	561	18	70	22	5	873
Roux (2 tsp. per serving)	12	106	1	8	8	---	61
Baked Salmon in Pastry	8	364	27	24	17	1	370
Catfish Piccata	4	327	21	15	16	2	954
Ginger Barbecue Salmon	6	272	30	4	14	---	384
Grilled Salmon Steak Sandwiches	4	412	30	39	14	3	1,017
Mustard Yogurt Dressing (3 tbsp. per serving)	4	65	2	2	4	---	393
Lobster Mac 'n' Cheese	4	685	41	64	29	3	1,048
Fresh Tomatillo Sauce (¼ cup per serving)	16	10	---	2	---	1	146

SEAFOOD (continued)	SERVINGS	CALORIES	PROTEIN (G)	CARBS (G)	FAT (G)	FIBER (G)	SODIUM (MG)
Miso & Maple–Marinated Cod	6	275	41	21	2	---	380
Sweet Pea Risotto	6	375	12	57	7	3	663
Pepper-Crusted Cod	4	278	42	7	8	1	712
Sambal (2 tbsp. per serving)	8	46	2	8	2	2	394

PORK

	SERVINGS	CALORIES	PROTEIN (G)	CARBS (G)	FAT (G)	FIBER (G)	SODIUM (MG)
Allen's Ramen (includes Quick Broth and Shoyu Base, Ramen Noodles)	4	847	62	119	13	6	5,384
Quick Broth	4	40	9	2	---	---	1,036
Ramen Noodles	4	495	16	99	2	3	305
Shoyu Base for Ramen	8	54	3	12	---	---	2,043
Slow Broth	24	24	1	---	2	---	7
Blackened Pork Loin	6	169	32	1	3	1	125
Baked Apples	6	76	---	15	2	1	194
Pickled Onions	6	13	---	3	---	1	197
Vindaloo Spice Mix (1 tbsp. per serving)	40	15	---	3	---	3	123
Country-Style Hoisin Ribs	6	456	40	28	18	---	2,706
Grilled Pork Chops	6	444	48	8	22	---	2,206
Kabocha Squash Mash	6	125	1	22	5	3	395
Basic Grilling Salt (1 tsp. per serving)	31	3	---	1	---	---	1,810
Roast Pork Loin with Peach Glaze	6	249	33	10	7	---	1,885
White Beans	6	100	4	16	3	3	234
Santa Fe Mac 'n' Cheese	4	473	29	65	11	8	588
Fresh Jalapeño Hot Sauce (1 tbsp. per serving)	8	7	---	---	---	---	291
Sausage, Potato & Kale Soup	6	463	22	38	26	7	1,304
Stewed Black-Eyed Peas with Salt Pork	6	462	9	22	38	6	1,172

BEEF LAMB BISON

	SERVINGS	CALORIES	PROTEIN (G)	CARBS (G)	FAT (G)	FIBER (G)	SODIUM (MG)
Beef & Beet Meatloaf	6	296	21	12	18	1	845
Bison Stew with Barley & Belgian Beer	8	330	31	31	8	6	826
Flank Steak with Torn Heirloom Tomatoes	6	308	34	8	15	2	1,370
Radish & Leek Slaw	6	15	---	4	---	---	395

BEEF LAMB BISON (continued)	SERVINGS	CALORIES	PROTEIN (G)	CARBS (G)	FAT (G)	FIBER (G)	SODIUM (MG)
Grilled T-Bones	4	532	76	1	25	---	779
Blue Cheese Dressing (1 tbsp. per serving)	4	24	1	2	1	---	224
Radicchio Slaw	4	113	3	4	10	1	514
Irish Lamb Stew with Guinness	8	272	28	21	7	3	803
Soda Bread	8	279	10	53	2	2	569
Lamb Chops	6	299	39	---	13	---	958
Cherry Jam (3 tbsp. per serving)	8	118	---	30	---	1	2
Farro	6	307	9	43	10	4	401
Fennel Slaw	6	27	1	6	---	2	51
Mac 'n' Cheese Bolognese	6	618	29	40	34	3	731

MEATLESS

	SERVINGS	CALORIES	PROTEIN (G)	CARBS (G)	FAT (G)	FIBER (G)	SODIUM (MG)
Baked Ziti with Toasted Chickpeas & Squash	4	375	16	44	15	8	784
Caviar Lentils	6	139	9	21	3	6	500
Chilled Soba with Spicy Red Beans & Poached Eggs	4	360	18	50	10	9	2,702
Eggplant & Onion Fried Wild Rice	4	442	20	68	11	8	410
Falafel (with pita and greens)	4	417	14	51	18	7	649
Chunky Cucumber Yogurt Sauce (½ cup per serving)	4	102	2	4	9	---	401
Homemade Egg Pasta	4	392	15	48	15	2	188
Fresh-Chopped Sauce (¼ cup per serving)	4	137	3	3	14	---	242
Mixed Bean Curry	6	452	18	58	17	17	635
Sweet Potato, Pecan & Mushroom "Meatloaf"	8	321	8	25	22	5	416

SWEET

	SERVINGS	CALORIES	PROTEIN (G)	CARBS (G)	FAT (G)	FIBER (G)	SODIUM (MG)
Almond Cornbread	8	430	14	54	19	7	376
Grilled Stone Fruit	8	79	1	12	4	2	---
Baked Granola Crisp (includes Homemade Granola)	6	367	4	69	10	4	61
Homemade Granola	6	304	4	55	9	3	10
Baklava	10	429	5	27	36	2	113
Banana Mousse Dessert	4	306	8	41	15	5	42

SWEET (continued)	SERVINGS	CALORIES	PROTEIN (G)	CARBS (G)	FAT (G)	FIBER (G)	SODIUM (MG)
Cashew Honey Brittle	8	338	5	46	17	1	390
Cinnamon Shortbread Cookies	10	358	5	46	18	2	102
Fresh Jam (2 tbsp. per serving)	10	38	---	10	---	2	1
Dark Chocolate Bark with Spiced Pumpkin Seeds	8	412	10	22	38	6	385
PB&J Cookies	10	467	6	48	29	2	185

Sauces Spices Oils Dressings

	SERVINGS	CALORIES	PROTEIN (G)	CARBS (G)	FAT (G)	FIBER (G)	SODIUM (MG)
Adacherri (2 tbsp.)	8	28	---	3	2	1	292
Balsamic Dipping Oil (1 tbsp.)	8	125	---	1	14	---	1
Blue Cheese Dressing (1 tbsp.)	4	24	1	2	1	---	224
Bright & Chunky Marinara (¾ cup)	4	186	5	27	8	7	528
Cherry Jam (3 tbsp.)	8	118	---	30	---	1	2
Chunky Cucumber Yogurt Sauce (½ cup)	4	102	2	4	9	---	401
Dijon Dressing (1 tbsp.)	6	83	---	---	9	---	158
Fresh-Chopped Sauce (1 tbsp.)	6	91	2	2	9	---	161
Fresh Jalapeño Hot Sauce (1 tbsp.)	8	7	---	---	---	---	291
Fresh Jam (2 tbsp.)	10	38	---	10	---	2	1
Fresh Tomatillo Sauce (¼ cup)	16	10	---	2	---	1	146
Ginger Barbecue Sauce (2 tbsp.)	6	18	---	4	---	---	123
Harissa (2 tbsp.)	12	87	2	9	6	4	202
Hoisin Sauce (¼ cup)	6	151	2	28	3	---	798
Homemade Barbecue Sauce (2 tbsp.)	16	32	---	8	---	1	185
Lemon Pesto (1 tbsp.)	16	92	1	1	10	---	42
Lemon Tarragon Dressing (1 tbsp.)	8	37	---	2	3	---	73
Mustard Yogurt Dressing (3 tbsp.)	4	65	2	2	4	---	393
Red Pepper Oil (1 tbsp.)	6	46	---	1	5	---	98
Red Pepper Sesame Oil Dressing (¼ cup)	4	129	---	2	14	1	586
Roasted Tomato Yogurt Sauce (¼ cup)	12	44	2	4	3	---	126
Sambal (2 tbsp.)	16	23	1	4	1	1	197
Yogurt Sauce (2 tbsp.)	6	33	2	3	1	---	75
Yuzu Dressing (2 tbsp.)	6	51	---	2	5	---	78

NOTES

1   A. Maslow and A. Herzeberg, "Hierarchy of Needs," in *Motivation and Personality*, ed. A. Maslow (New York: Harper, 1954).

2   H. F. Harlow, "The Nature of Love," *American Psychologist* 13, no. 12 (December 1958): 673.

3   H. D. Chapin, "Are Institutions for Infants Necessary?" *Journal of the American Medical Association* 64, no. 1 (January 1915): 1–3.

4   P. H. Gray, "Henry Dwight Chapin: Pioneer in the Study of Institutionalized Infants," *Bulletin of the Psychonomic Society* 27, no. 1 (January 1989): 85–87.

5   J. Williamson and A. Greenberg, *Families, Not Orphanages* (New York: Better Care Network, 2010).

6   D. Tobis, *Moving from Residential Institutions to Community-Based Social Services in Central and Eastern Europe and the Former Soviet Union* (Washington, DC: The World Bank, 2000).

7   M. H. Van Ijzendoorn, M. P. C. M. Luijk, and F. Juffer, "IQ of Children Growing Up in Children's Homes: A Meta-Analysis on IQ Delays in Orphanages," *Merrill-Palmer Quarterly* 54 (2008): 341–66.

8   S. Achor, *The Happiness Advantage: The Seven Principles of Positive Psychology That Fuel Success and Performance at Work* (New York: Random House, 2011).

9   R. Wimmer, "Elite Athletes and Treating Post-Competition Depression," *Sports Medicine* 11 (2003): 12–15.

10 C. Fischler, "Commensality, Society and Culture," *Social Science Information* 50, no. 3–4 (2011): 528–48.

11 http://dictionary.reference.com/browse/mensa?s=t.

12 A. A. Barb, "Mensa Sacra: The Round Table and the Holy Grail," *Journal of the Warburg and Courtauld Institutes* 19, no. 1–2 (1956): 40–67.

13 T. L. Bray, ed., *The Archaeology and Politics of Food and Feasting in Early States and Empires* (New York: Springer, 2003); R. Wrangham, Catching Fire: How Cooking Made Us Human (New York: Basic Books, 2009); S. Kerner, C. Chou, and M. Warmind, eds., *Commensality: From Everyday Food to Feast* (New York: Bloomsbury, 2015).

14 P. G. W. Glare, *Oxford Latin Dictionary* (Oxford: Oxford University Press, 1982).

15 B. Hare and S. Kwetuenda, "Bonobos Voluntarily Share Their Own Food with Others," *Current Biology* 20, no. 5 (March 2010): R230–31.

16 L. Miller, P. Rozin, and A. P. Fiske, "Food Sharing and Feeding Another Person Suggest Intimacy: Two Studies of American College Students," *European Journal of Social Psychology* 28 (1998): 423–36.

17 K. M. Kniffin and B. Wansink, "It's Not Just Lunch: Extra-Pair Commensality Can Trigger Sexual Jealousy," *Plos One* 7 (July 2012): E40445.

18 S. Mennell, A. Murcott, and A. Van Otterloo, "Conclusion: Commensality and Society," *Current Sociology* 40, no. 2 (September 1992): 115–19; C. M. Counihan, "Food Rules in the United States: Control, Hierarchy and Individualism," *Anthropological Quarterly* 65, no. 2 (April 1992): 55–66.

19 A. Murcott, "Family Meals: A Thing of the Past," in *Food, Health and Identity*, ed. Pat Caplan (New York: Rutledge, 1997), 32–49.

20 A. Murcott, "Lamenting 'the Decline of the Family Meal' as a Moral Panic? Methodological Reflections," *Recherches Sociologiques et Anthropologiques* 43, no. 1 (2012): 97–118.

21 D. Neumark-Sztainer, M. E. Eisenberg, J. A. Fulkerson, M. Story, and N. I. Larson, "Family Meals and Disordered Eating in Adolescents: Longitudinal Findings from Project Eat," *Archives of Pediatrics & Adolescent Medicine* 162, no. 1 (2008): 17–22; J. A. Fulkerson, M. Story, A. Mellin, N. Leffert, D. Neumark-Sztainer, and S. A. French, "Family Dinner Meal Frequency and Adolescent Development: Relationships with Developmental Assets and High-Risk Behaviors," *Journal of Adolescent Health* 39, no. 3 (September 2006): 337–45.

22 E. M. Taveras, S. L. Rifas Shiman, C. S. Berkey, H. R. H. Rockett, A. E. Field, A. L. Frazier, G. A. Colditz, and M. W. Gillman, "Family Dinner and Adolescent Overweight," *Obesity Research* 13, no. 5 (May 2005): 900–6.

23 B. Sen, "Frequency of Family Dinner and Adolescent Body Weight Status: Evidence from the National Longitudinal Survey of Youth, 1997," *Obesity* 14, no. 12 (December 2006): 2266–76.

24 J. Sobal and M. K. Nelson, "Commensal Eating Patterns: A Community Study," *Appetite* 41, no. 2 (October 2003): 181–90.

25 A. Murcott, "Family Meals: A Thing of the Past," in *Food, Health and Identity*, ed. Pat Caplan (New York; Routledge, 1997): 32–49.

26 D. Neumark-Sztainer, M. Wall, J. A. Fulkerson, and N. Larson, "Changes in the Frequency of Family Meals from 1999 to 2010 in the Homes of Adolescents: Trends by Sociodemographic Characteristics," *Journal of Adolescent Health* 52, no. 2 (February 2013): 201–6.

27 J. White and E. Halliwell, "Alcohol and Tobacco Use During Adolescence: The Importance of the Family Mealtime Environment," *Journal of Health Psychology* 15, no. 4 (May 2010): 526–32.

28 S. Sierra-Baigrie, S. Lemos-Giráldez, and E. Fonseca-Pedrero, "Binge Eating in Adolescents: Its Relation to Behavioural Problems and Family-Meal Patterns," *Eating Behaviors* 10, no. 1 (February 2009): 22–28.

29 S. J. Woodruff and R. M. Hanning, "Associations Between Family Dinner Frequency and Specific Food Behaviors Among Grade Six, Seven, and Eight Students from Ontario and Nova Scotia," *Journal of Adolescent Health* 44, no. 5 (June 2009): 431–36.

30 F. Bellisle and M. F. Rolland Cachera, "Three Consecutive (1993, 1995, 1997) Surveys of Food Intake, Nutritional Attitudes and Knowledge, and Lifestyle in 1,000 French Children, Aged 9–11 Years," *Journal of Human Nutrition and Dietetics* 13, no. 2 (April 2000): 101–11.

31 M. E. Harrison, M. L. Norris, N. Obeid, M. Fu, H. Weinstangel, and M. Sampson, "Systematic Review of the Effects of Family Meal Frequency on Psychosocial Outcomes in Youth," *Canadian Family Physician* 61, no. 2 (February 2015): E96–106.

32 H. Patrick and T. A. Nicklas, "A Review of Family and Social Determinants of Children's Eating Patterns and Diet Quality," *Journal of the American College of Nutrition* 24, no. 2 (April 2005): 83–92.

33 T. L. Burgess-Champoux, N. Larson, D. Neumark-Sztainer, P. J. Hannan, and M. Story, "Are Family Meal Patterns Associated with Overall Diet Quality During the Transition from Early to Middle Adolescence?" *Journal of Nutrition Education and Behavior* 41, no. 2 (March/April 2009): 79–86.

34 N. I. Larson, D. Neumark-Sztainer, P. J. Hannan, and M. Story, "Family Meals During Adolescence Are Associated with Higher Diet Quality and Healthful Meal Patterns During Young Adulthood," *Journal of the American Dietetic Association* 107, no. 9 (September 2007): 1502–10; A. J. Hammons and B. H. Fiese, "Is Frequency of Shared Family Meals Related to the Nutritional Health of Children and Adolescents?" *Pediatrics* 127, no. 6 (June 2011): E1565–74; C. J. De Backer, "Family Meal Traditions: Comparing Reported Childhood Food Habits to Current Food Habits Among University Students," *Appetite* 69 (October 2013): 64–70.

35 V. Skafida, "The Family Meal Panacea: Exploring How Different Aspects of Family Meal Occurrence, Meal Habits and Meal Enjoyment Relate to Young Children's Diets," *Sociology of Health and Illness* 35, no. 6 (July 2013): 906–23.

36 A. J. Hammons and B. H. Fiese, "Is Frequency of Shared Family Meals Related to the Nutritional Health

of Children and Adolescents?" *Pediatrics* 127, no. 6 (June 2011): E1565–74.

37 E. M Taveras, S. L. Rifas Shiman, C. S. Berkey, H. R. H. Rockett, A. E. Field, A. L. Frazier, G. A. Colditz, and M. W. Gillman, "Family Dinner and Adolescent Overweight," *Obesity Research* 13, no. 5 (May 2005): 900–6.

38 B. Sen, "Frequency of Family Dinner and Adolescent Body Weight Status: Evidence from the National Longitudinal Survey of Youth, 1997," *Obesity* 14, no. 12 (December 2006): 2266–76.

39 J. A. Fulkerson, N. Larson, M. Horning, and D. Neumark-Sztainer, "A Review of Associations Between Family or Shared Meal Frequency and Dietary and Weight Status Outcomes Across the Lifespan," *Journal of Nutrition Education and Behavior* 46, no. 1 (January 2014): 2–19.

40 D. L. Franko, D. Thompson, R. Bauserman, S. G. Affenito, and R. H. Striegel Moore, "What's Love Got to Do with It? Family Cohesion and Healthy Eating Behaviors in Adolescent Girls," *International Journal of Eating Disorders* 41, no. 4 (May 2008): 360–67; D. Neumark-Sztainer, M. Wall, M. Story, and J. A. Fulkerson, "Are Family Meal Patterns Associated with Disordered Eating Behaviors Among Adolescents?" *Journal of Adolescent Health* 35, no. 5 (November 2004): 350–59; D. Neumark-Sztainer, M. E. Eisenberg, J. A. Fulkerson, M. Story, and N. I. Larson, "Family Meals and Disordered Eating in Adolescents: Longitudinal Findings from Project Eat," *Archives of Pediatrics & Adolescent Medicine* 162, no. 1 (January 2008): 17–22; M. Mateos-Agut, I. García-Alonso, J. J. De La Gándara-Martín, M. I. Vegas-Miguel, C. Sebastián-Vega, B. Sanz-Cid, A. Martínez-Villares, and E. Martín-Martínez, "Family Structure and Eating Behavior Disorders," *Actas Españolas de Psiquiatría* 42, no. 6 (November/December 2014): 267–80.

41 J. White and E. Halliwell, "Alcohol and Tobacco Use During Adolescence: The Importance of the Family Mealtime Environment," *Journal of Health Psychology* 15, no. 4 (May 2010): 526–32; M. E. Eisenberg, D. Neumark-Sztainer, J. A. Fulkerson, and M. Story, "Family Meals and Substance Use: Is There a Long-Term Protective Association?" *Journal of Adolescent Health* 43, no. 2 (August 2008): 151–56; J. A. Fulkerson, M. Story, A. Mellin, N. Leffert, D. Neumark-Sztainer, and S. A. French, "Family Dinner Meal Frequency and Adolescent Development:

Relationships with Developmental Assets and High-Risk Behaviors," *Journal of Adolescent Health* 39, no. 3 (September 2006): 337–45.

42 J. R. Ickovics, A. Carroll-Scott, S. M. Peters, M. Schwartz, K. Gilstad-Hayden, and C. McCaslin, "Health and Academic Achievement: Cumulative Effects of Health Assets on Standardized Test Scores Among Urban Youth in the United States," *Journal of School Health* 84, no. 1 (January 2014): 40–48.

43 K. Loth, M. Wall, C. W. Choi, M. Bucchianeri, V. Quick, N. Larson, and D. Neumark-Sztainer, "Family Meals and Disordered Eating in Adolescents: Are the Benefits the Same for Everyone?" *International Journal of Eating Disorders* 48, no. 1 (January 2015): 100–10.

44 J. A. Fulkerson, K. E. Pasch, M. H. Stigler, K. Farbakhsh, C. L. Perry, and K. A. Komro, "Longitudinal Associations Between Family Dinner and Adolescent Perceptions of Parent-Child Communication Among Racially Diverse Urban Youth," *Journal of Family Psychology* 24, no. 3 (June 2010): 261.

45 M. Tomasello, *Why We Cooperate* (Cambridge, MA: MIT Press, 2009).

46 http://www.who.int/topics/cardiovascular_diseases/en/.

47 K. M. Anderson, P. M. Odell, P. W. F. Wilson, and W. B. Kannel, "Cardiovascular Disease Risk Profiles," *American Heart Journal* 121, no. 1 (January 1991): 293–98.

48 A. Mente, L. De Koning, H. S. Shannon, and S. S. Anand, "A Systematic Review of the Evidence Supporting a Causal Link Between Dietary Factors and Coronary Heart Disease," *Archives of Internal Medicine* 169, no. 7 (April 2009): 659–69.

49 T. A. Pearson, S. N. Blair, S. R. Daniels, R. H. Eckel, J. M. Fair, S. P. Fortmann, B. A. Franklin, L. B. Goldstein, P. Greenland, and S. M. Grundy, "AHA Guidelines for Primary Prevention of Cardiovascular Disease and Stroke: 2002 Update Consensus Panel Guide to Comprehensive Risk Reduction for Adult Patients Without Coronary or Other Atherosclerotic Vascular Diseases," *Circulation* 106 (2002): 388–91; M. J. Stampfer, F. B. Hu, J. E. Manson, E. B. Rimm, and W. C. Willett, "Primary Prevention of Coronary Heart Disease in Women Through Diet and Lifestyle," *New England Journal of Medicine* 343 (July 2000): 16–22.

50 J. Ferrières, "The French Paradox: Lessons for Other Countries," *Heart* 90, no. 1 (January 2004): 107–11.

51 J. A. Negold, P. Asaria, and D. P. Francis, "Mortality from Ischaemic Heart Disease by Country, Region, and Age: Statistics from World Health Organisation and United Nations," *International Journal of Cardiology* 168, no. 2 (September 2013): 934–45.

52 R. Masiá, A. Pena, J. Marrugat, J. Sala, J. Vila, M. Pavesi, M. Covas, C. Aubó, and R. Elosua, "High Prevalence of Cardiovascular Risk Factors in Gerona, Spain, a Province with Low Myocardial Infarction Incidence. REGICOR Investigators," *Journal of Epidemiology and Community Health* 52, no. 11 (November 1998): 707–15.

53 J. Ferrières, "The French Paradox: Lessons for Other Countries," *Heart* 90, no. 1 (January 2004): 107–11; A. Drewnowski, S. A. Henderson, A. Shore, C. Fischler, P. Preziosi, and S. Hercberg, "Diet Quality and Dietary Diversity in France: Implications for the French Paradox," *Journal of the American Dietetic Association* 96, no. 6 (July 1996): 663–69.

54 P. Rozin, A. K. Remick, and C. Fischler, "Broad Themes of Difference Between French and Americans in Attitudes to Food and Other Life Domains: Personal Versus Communal Values, Quantity Versus Quality, and Comforts Versus Joys," *Frontiers in Psychology* 2 (2011); P. Rozin, C. Fischler, C. Sheilds, and E. Masson, "Attitudes Towards Large Numbers of Choices in the Food Domain: A Cross-Cultural Study of Five Countries in Europe and the USA," *Appetite* 46, no. 3 (May 2011): 304–8; R. Eckersley, "Is Modern Western Culture a Health Hazard?" *International Journal of Epidemiology* 35, no. 2 (April 2006): 252–58; P. Rozin, C. Fischler, S. Imada, A. Sarubin, and A. Wrzesniewski, "Attitudes to Food and the Role of Food in Life in the USA, Japan, Flemish Belgium and France: Possible Implications for the Diet-Health Debate," *Appetite* 33, no. 2 (October 1999): 163–80.

55 P. Rozin, K. Kabnick, E. Pete, C. Fischler, and C. Shields, "The Ecology of Eating: Smaller Portion Sizes in France Than in the United States Helps Explain the French Paradox," *Psychological Science* 14, no. 5 (September 2003): 450–54.

56 L. Hedegaard, "Food Studies in French History: French Meals: Commensality, Synchronisation and Structure," *Society for French Historical Studies* (November 2011); J. Riou, T. Lefèvre, I. Parizot, A. Lhuissier, and P. Chauvin, "Is There Still a French Eating Model? A Taxonomy of Eating Behaviors in Adults Living in the Paris Metropolitan Area in 2010," *Plos One* 10, no. 3 (March 2015): E0119161; S. Gojard, "Meal Schedules in Early Childhood: A Study in Contemporary France," *Food and Foodways* 9, no. 3–4 (April 2001): 187–203.

57 N. A. Christakis and J. H. Fowler, "Social Contagion Theory: Examining Dynamic Social Networks and Human Behavior," *Statistics in Medicine* 32, no. 4 (February 2013): 556–77.

58 M. Laroche, I. Takahashi, M. Kalamas, and L. Teng, "Modeling the Selection of Fast-Food Franchises Among Japanese Consumers," *Journal of Business Research* 58, no. 8 (August 2005): 1121–31.

59 M. A. Pereira, A. I. Kartashov, C. B. Ebbeling, L. Van Horn, M. L. Slattery, D. R. Jacobs, and D. S. Ludwig, "Fast-Food Habits, Weight Gain, and Insulin Resistance (The Cardia Study): 15-Year Prospective Analysis," *The Lancet* 365, no. 9453 (January 2005): 36–42; D. A. Alter and K. Eny, "The Relationship Between the Supply of Fast-Food Chains and Cardiovascular Outcomes," *Canadian Journal of Public Health* 96, no. 3 (May–June 2005): 173–77; S. A. Bowman, S. L. Gortmaker, C. B. Ebbeling, M. A. Pereira, and D. S. Ludwig, "Effects of Fast-Food Consumption on Energy Intake and Diet Quality Among Children in a National Household Survey," Pediatrics 113 (January 2004): 112–18; B. Fortin and M. Yazbeck, "Peer Effects, Fast Food Consumption and Adolescent Weight Gain," *Journal of Health Economics* 42 (July 2015): 125–38.

60 J. Boone-Heinonen, P. Gordon-Larsen, C. I. Kiefe, J. M. Shikany, C. E. Lewis, and B. M. Popkin, "Fast Food Restaurants and Food Stores: Longitudinal Associations with Diet in Young- to Middle-Aged Adults: The CARDIA Study," *Archives of Internal Medicine* 171, no. 13 (July 2011): 1162–70; K. W. Bauer, N. I. Larson, M. C. Nelson, M. Story, and D. Neumark-Sztainer, "Socio-Environmental, Personal and Behavioural Predictors of Fast-Food Intake Among Adolescents," *Public Health Nutrition* 12, no. 10 (October 2009): 1767–74.

61 https://en.wikipedia.org/wiki/Anomie.

62 J. W. Traphagan and L. K. Brown, "Fast Food and Intergenerational Commensality in Japan: New Styles

and Old Patterns," *Ethnology* 41, no. 2 (2002): 119–34.

63 J. L. Derrick, S. Gabriel, and K. Hugenberg, "Social Surrogacy: How Favored Television Programs Provide the Experience of Belonging," *Journal of Experimental Social Psychology* 45, no. 2 (February 2009): 352–62.

64 J. D. Troisi and S. Gabriel, "Chicken Soup Really Is Good for the Soul: 'Comfort Food' Fulfills the Need to Belong," *Psychological Science* 22 (April 2011): 747–53.

65 C. E. Moustakas, *Loneliness* (Englewood Cliffs, NJ: Prentice-Hall, 1961).

66 www.ted.com/talks/guy_winch_the_case_for_emotional_hygiene?language=en.

67 E. B. Loucks, L. M. Sullivan, R. B. D'Agostino, M. G. Larson, L. F. Berkman, and E. J. Benjamin, "Social Networks and Inflammatory Markers in the Framingham Heart Study," *Journal of Biosocial Science* 38, no. 6 (November 2006): 835–42; D. Sorkin, K. S. Rook, and J. L. Lu, "Loneliness, Lack of Emotional Support, Lack of Companionship, and the Likelihood of Having a Heart Condition in an Elderly Sample," *Annals of Behavioral Medicine* 24, no. 4 (2002): 290–98.

68 C. McCrory, C. Finucane, C. O'Hare, J. Frewen, H. Nolan, R. Layte, P. M. Kearney, and R. A. Kenny, "Social Disadvantage and Social Isolation Are Associated with a Higher Resting Heart Rate: Evidence from the Irish Longitudinal Study on Ageing," *The Journals of Gerontology Series B: Psychological Sciences and Social Sciences* (December 2014).

69 R. C. Thurston and L. D. Kubzansky, "Women, Loneliness, and Incident Coronary Heart Disease," *Psychosomatic Medicine* 71, no. 8 (October 2009): 836–42.

70 V. Yiengprugsawan, C. Banwell, W. Takeda, J. Dixon, S. A. Seubsman, and A. C. Sleigh, "Health, Happiness and Eating Together: What Can a Large Thai Cohort Study Tell Us?" *Global Journal of Health Science* 7, no. 4 (2015): 42114; J. T. Cacioppo, J. H. Fowler, and N. A. Christakis, "Alone in the Crowd: The Structure and Spread of Loneliness in a Large Social Network," *Journal of Personality and Social Psychology* 97, no. 6 (December 2009): 977–91.

71 C. Löfvenmark, A. C. Mattiasson, E. Billing, and M. Edner, "Perceived Loneliness and Social Support in Patients with Chronic Heart Failure," *European Journal of Cardiovascular Nursing* 8, no. 4 (October 2009): 251–58.

72 J. Geller, P. Janson, E. McGovern, and A. Valdini, "Loneliness as a Predictor of Hospital Emergency Department Use," *The Journal of Family Practice* 48, no. 12 (December 1999): 801–4.

73 J. Crossman and J. Jamieson, "Differences in Perceptions of Seriousness and Disrupting Effects of Athletic Injury as Viewed by Athletes and Their Trainer," *Perceptual and Motor Skills* 61, no. 3, pt. 2 (December 1985): 1131–34.

74 J. Tomaka, S. Thompson, and R. Palacios, "The Relation of Social Isolation, Loneliness, and Social Support to Disease Outcomes Among the Elderly," *Journal of Aging and Health* 18, no. 3 (June 2006): 359–84.

75 A. C. Patterson and G. Veenstra, "Loneliness and Risk of Mortality: A Longitudinal Investigation in Alameda County, California," *Social Science and Medicine* 71, no. 1 (July 2010): 181–86.

76 R. M. Cawthon, K. R. Smith, E. O'Brien, A. Sivatchenko, and R. A. Kerber, "Association Between Telomere Length in Blood and Mortality in People Aged 60 Years or Older," *The Lancet* 361, no. 9355 (February 2003): 393–95; E. S. Epel, S. S. Merkin, R. Cawthon, E. H. Blackburn, N. E. Adler, M. J. Pletcher, and T. E. Seeman, "The Rate of Leukocyte Telomere Shortening Predicts Mortality from Cardiovascular Disease in Elderly Men," *Aging* 1, no. 1 (January 2009): 81–88.

77 J. E. Carroll, A. V. Diez Roux, A. L. Fitzpatrick, and T. Seeman, "Low Social Support Is Associated with Shorter Leukocyte Telomere Length in Late Life: Multi-Ethnic Study of Atherosclerosis," *Psychosomatic Medicine* 75, no. 2 (February 2013): 171–77.

78 A. Shankar, M. Hamer, A. McMunn, and A. Steptoe, "Social Isolation and Loneliness: Relationships with Cognitive Function During 4 Years of Follow-Up in the English Longitudinal Study of Ageing," *Psychosomatic Medicine* 75, no. 2 (February 2013): 161–70.

79 E. Ramic, N. Pranjic, O. Batic-Mujanovic, E. Karic, E. Alibasic, and A. Alic, "The Effect of Loneliness on Malnutrition in Elderly Population," *Medical*

Archives 65, no. 2 (2011): 92–95; G. Hughes, K. M. Bennett, and M. M. Hetherington, "Old and Alone: Barriers to Healthy Eating in Older Men Living on Their Own," *Appetite* 43, no. 3 (December 2004): 269–76; Y. Tani, N. Kondo, D. Takagi, M. Saito, H. Hikichi, T. Ojima, and K. Kondo, "Combined Effects of Eating Alone and Living Alone on Unhealthy Dietary Behaviors, Obesity and Underweight in Older Japanese Adults: Results of the JAGES," *Appetite* 95 (December 2015): 1–8.

80 L. Wright, L. Vance, C. Sudduth, and J. B. Epps, "The Impact of a Home-Delivered Meal Program on Nutritional Risk, Dietary Intake, Food Security, Loneliness, and Social Well-Being," *Journal of Nutrition in Gerontology and Geriatrics* 34, no. 2 (2015): 218–27.

81 M. P. Levine, "Loneliness and Eating Disorders," *Journal of Health Psychology* 146, no. 1–2 (January–April 2012): 243–57.

82 J. Sundgot-Borgen and M. K. Torstveit, "Prevalence of Eating Disorders in Elite Athletes Is Higher Than in the General Population," *Clinical Journal of Sport Medicine* 14, no. 1 (January 2004): 25–32.

83 S. Byrne and N. McLean, "Eating Disorders in Athletes: A Review of the Literature," *Journal of Science and Medicine in Sport* 4, no. 2 (June 2001): 145–59.

84 A. Rokach, "Loneliness Then and Now: Reflections on Social and Emotional Alienation in Everyday Life," *Current Psychology* 23, no. 1 (March 2004): 24–40; A. Rokach, "Perceived Causes of Loneliness in Adulthood," *Journal of Social Behavior and Personality* 15, no. 1 (March 2000): 67.

85 V. Yiengprugsawan, C. Banwell, W. Takeda, J. Dixon, S. A. Seubsman, and A. C. Sleigh, "Health, Happiness and Eating Together: What Can a Large Thai Cohort Study Tell Us?" *Global Journal of Health Science* 7, no. 4 (2015): 42114.

86 A. Kuroda, T. Tanaka, H. Hirano, Y. Ohara, T. Kikutani, H. Furuya, S. P. Obuchi, H. Kawai, S. Ishii, M. Akishita, T. Tsuji, and K. Iijima, "Eating Alone as Social Disengagement Is Strongly Associated with Depressive Symptoms in Japanese Community-Dwelling Older Adults," *Journal of the American Medical Directors Association* 16, no. 7 (July 2015): 578–85; P. Pliner and R. Bell, "A Table for One: The Pain and Pleasure of Eating Alone," in *Meals in Science and Practice: Interdisciplinary Research and Business Applications*, ed. H. L. Meiselman (Cambridge: CRD Press & Woodhead, 2009), 169–89.

87 P. Pliner and R. Bell, "A Table for One: The Pain and Pleasure of Eating Alone," in *Meals in Science and Practice: Interdisciplinary Research and Business Applications*, ed. H. L. Meiselman (Cambridge: CRD Press & Woodhead, 2009), 169–89.

88 J. T. Cacioppo and W. Patrick, *Loneliness: Human Nature and the Need for Social Connection* (New York: W. W. Norton, 2009).

89 S. Bofill, "Aging and Loneliness in Catalonia: The Social Dimension of Food Behavior," *Ageing International* 29, no. 4 (December 2004): 385–98.

90 R. Larson, M. Csikszentmihalyi, and R. Graef, "Time Alone in Daily Experience: Loneliness or Renewal," in *Loneliness: A Sourcebook of Current Theory, Research and Therapy*, ed. Letitia Anne Peplau and Daniel Perlman (New York: Wiley, 1982), 40–53.

91 N. A. Christakis and J. H. Fowler, "Social Contagion Theory: Examining Dynamic Social Networks and Human Behavior," *Statistics in Medicine* 32, no. 4 (February 2013): 556–77.

92 J. T. Cacioppo, J. H. Fowler, and N. A. Christakis, "Alone in the Crowd: The Structure and Spread of Loneliness in a Large Social Network," *Journal of Personality and Social Psychology* 97, no. 6 (December 2009): 977–91.

93 J. N. Rosenquist, J. H. Fowler, and N. A. Christakis, "Social Network Determinants of Depression," *Molecular Psychiatry* 16 (2011): 273–81; N. A. Christakis and J. H. Fowler, "The Collective Dynamics of Smoking in a Large Social Network," *New England Journal of Medicine* 358 (May 2008): 2249–58; R. McDermott, J. Fowler, and N. Christakis, "Breaking Up Is Hard to Do, Unless Everyone Else Is Doing It Too: Social Network Effects on Divorce in a Longitudinal Sample," *Social Forces* 92, no. 2 (December 2013): 491–519; J. N. Rosenquist, J. Murabito, J. H. Fowler, and N. A. Christakis, "The Spread of Alcohol Consumption Behavior in a Large Social Network," *Annals of Internal Medicine* 152, no. 7 (April 2010): 426–33, W141; N. A. Christakis and J. H. Fowler, "The Spread of Obesity in a Large Social Network over 32 Years," *New England*

Journal of Medicine 357 (July 2007): 370–79; P. A. Quatromoni, D. L. Copenhafer, S. Demissie, R. B. D'Agostino, C. E. O'Horo, B. H. Nam, and B. E. Millen, "The Internal Validity of a Dietary Pattern Analysis: The Framingham Nutrition Studies," *Journal of Epidemiology and Community Health* 56, no. 5 (May 2002): 381–88; B. E. Millen, P. A. Quatromoni, D. L. Copenhafer, S. Demissie, C. E. O'Horo, and R. B. D'Agostino, "Validation of a Dietary Pattern Approach or Evaluating Nutritional Risk: The Framingham Nutrition Studies," *Journal of the Academy of Nutrition and Dietetics* 101, no. 2 (February 2001): 187–94; M. A. Pachucki, P. F. Jacques, and N. A. Christakis, "Social Network Concordance in Food Choice Among Spouses, Friends, and Siblings," *American Journal of Public Health* 101, no. 11 (November 2011): 2170–77; A. J. O'Malley and N. A. Christakis, "Longitudinal Analysis of Large Social Networks: Estimating the Effect of Health Traits on Changes in Friendship Ties," *Statistics in Medicine* 30, no. 9 (April 2011): 950–64.

94 J. H. Fowler and N. A. Christakis, "Dynamic Spread of Happiness in a Large Social Network: Longitudinal Analysis over 20 Years in the Framingham Heart Study," *The BMJ* 337 (December 2008): A2338.

95 www.npr.org/2015/07/31/426842528/can-healthy-eating-reverse-some-cancers.

96 G. J. Armelagos, T. Leatherman, M. Ryan, and L. Sibley, "Biocultural Synthesis in Medical Anthropology," *Medical Anthropology* 14, no. 1 (March 1992): 35–52.

97 https://en.wikipedia.org/wiki/Soylent_%28drink%29.

98 R. Eckersley, "Is Modern Western Culture a Health Hazard?" *International Journal of Epidemiology* 35, no. 2 (April 2006): 252–58.

99 F. Crosby, "A Model of Egoistical Relative Deprivation," *Psychological Review* 83, no. 2 (March 1976): 85; M. Marmot and R. G. Wilkinson, "Psychosocial and Material Pathways in the Relation Between Income and Health: A Response to Lynch et al.," *The BMJ* 322 (May 2001): 1233; C. Eibner and W. N. Evans, "Relative Deprivation, Poor Health Habits, and Mortality," *Journal of Human Resources* 40, no. 3 (Summer 2005): 591–620.

100 R. Moynihan and A. Cassels, *Selling Sickness: How Drug Companies Are Turning Us into Patients* (New York: Nation Books, 2005), 254.

101 S. Woloshin and L. M. Schwartz, "Giving Legs to Restless Legs: A Case Study of How the Media Helps Make People Sick," *Plos Medicine* 3 (April 2006): 452.

102 H. Benson, "The Nocebo Effect: History and Physiology," *Preventive Medicine* 26, no. 5, pt. 1 (September 1997): 612–15; E. Carlino, A. Piedimonte, and E. Frisaldi, eds.,"The Effects of Placebos and Nocebos on Physical Performance," in *Placebo* (New York: Springer, 2014), 149–57.

103 J. Kim, R. Larose, and W. Peng, "Loneliness as the Cause and the Effect of Problematic Internet Use: The Relationship Between Internet Use and Psychological Well-Being," *Cyberpsychology & Behavior* 12, no. 4 (August 2009): 451–55.

104 Daniel Coyle, *The Talent Code: Greatness Isn't Born. It's Grown. Here's How.* (New York: Bantam, 2009).

105 L. Hallberg, L. Garby, R. Suwanik, and E. Bjorn-Rasmussen, "Iron Absorption from Southeast Asian Diets," *American Journal of Clinical Nutrition* 27, no. 8 (August 1974): 826–36.

106 L. Hallberg, E. Bjorn-Rasmussen, L. Rossander, and R. Suwanik, "Iron Absorption from Southeast Asian Diets, II. Role of Various Factors That Might Explain Low Absorption," *American Journal of Clinical Nutrition* 30, no. 4 (April 1977): 539–48.

107 R. H. Lustig, L. A. Schmidt, and C. D. Brindis, "Public Health: The Toxic Truth About Sugar," *Nature* 482 (February 2012): 27–29.

108 J. Belkova, M. Rozkot, P. Danek, P. Klein, J. Matonohova, and I. Podhorna, "Sugar and Nutritional Extremism," *Critical Reviews in Food Science and Nutrition* 21 (April 2015).

109 www.esquire.com/news-politics/a4310/the-crack-up.

INDEX

Note: Page numbers in italics refer to illustrations.

Adacherri, 115
Allen's Ramen, 221–222
Almond meal, 165, 281
Almond milk, 69, 238, 278
Almond Cornbread with Grilled Stone Fruit,
    280, 281
Anchovies, 83
Apples, 208, 56
Armstrong, Lance, 31–33
Artichokes, *72*, 73–74
Athletic performance
    eating alone and, 33–34
    Five-Ring Fever, 7
    goals, 7, 8, 9
    happiness versus success, 8–9
    loneliness and, 22, 23
    nocebo effect, 31
    training methodology, 5–7
Atkinson, Monte, 3
Avocados, 113, 77

Bacon
    Baked Jambalaya, 180, *181*
    Chicken & Almond Dumplings, *164*, 165
    Grilled Romaine with Pancetta, Hard-Boiled
        Eggs & Dijon Dressing, 123, *124*, 125
    Mac 'n' Cheese Bolognese, *240*, 241
    Spicy Red Beans & Rice, 118, *119*
    Stewed Black-Eyed Peas with Salt Pork,
        212, 213
Baked Apples, 208
Baked Biriyani, 170, *171*
Baked Chicken Parmesan with Bright & Chunky
    Marinara, *148*, 149–150

Baked Granola Crisp, 278, *279*
Baked Jambalaya, 180, *181*
Baked Salmon in Pastry, *190*, 191–192
Baked Ziti with Toasted Chickpeas & Squash, *256*, 257
Baklava, *284*, 285
Balsamic Dipping Oil, 73
Banana Mousse Dessert, 272, *273*
Barbecue sauce, homemade, 163
Barley, 243
Basic Grilling Salt, 206
Basil, 80, *79*
Bay scallops, 108
Beans
    Chilled Black Bean Yogurt Soup, 102, *103*
    Chilled Soba with Spicy Red Beans & Poached
        Eggs, 254, *255*
    cooking from dry, 280
    Guacamole with Beans, *79*, 80
    Mixed Bean Curry, *258*, 259
    Roast Pork Loin with Peach Glaze & White Beans,
        216, *217*
    Santa Fe Mac 'n' Cheese, *214*, 215
    Spicy Red Beans & Rice, 118, *119*
Beef
    Beef & Beet Meatloaf, *234*, 235
    Beef Bone Stock, 98–99
    Flank Steak with Torn Heirloom Tomatoes, *232*, 233
    Grilled T-Bones with Blue Cheese Dressing &
        Radicchio Slaw, *244*, 245, 246
    Mac 'n' Cheese Bolognese, *240*, 241
Beer, 243, 237–238
Beets
    Beef & Beet Meatloaf, *234*, 235
    Red Chicken with Baked Biriyani, 170, *171*
    Split Chicken with Lemon Garlic Sauce & Roasted
        Vegetables, 154, *155*

Bell peppers
    Baked Jambalaya, 180, *181*
    Bright & Chunky Marinara, 149
    Chilled Black Bean Yogurt Soup, 102, *103*
    Red Pepper Oil, 78, 137
Belonging, 2, 3, 6, 7, 21, 28
Biriyani, 170
Bison Stew with Barley & Belgian Beer, *242, 243*
Bitter Chard on Grilled Bread, 88, *89*
Blackened Pork Loin & Pickled Onions with Baked
    Apples, *207*, 208
Black-eyed peas, 213
Blue Cheese Dressing, 245
Bolognese, *240*, 241
Bread
    Bitter Chard on Grilled Bread, 88, *89*
    Grilled Bread & Artichokes with Dipping Oil,
    72, 73–74
    Soda Bread, *236, 237*–238
    Torn Bread & Radicchio Salad, 106, *107*
    White Anchovy Toast, *82*, 83
Bright & Chunky Marinara, 149–150
Broccoli Soup with Smoked Trout & Chives,
    116, 117
Broth, 121, 221, 222
Brussels sprouts, 154

Cabbage, 250
    Cabbage Slaw, 143
    Chilled Soba with Spicy Red Beans & Poached
    Eggs, *254, 255*
    Chopped Chicken Salad with Pickled Onions
    & Radishes, 147, *148*
    Citrus Salad with Yuzu Dressing & Wonton Crisps,
    128, *129*
    Kimchee Spiced Salad, *126*, 127
Cardiovascular disease, 17, 18–20, 24
Carrots, *See* Vegetables
Cashew Honey Brittle, *276, 277*
Catfish Piccata, 183
Cauliflower & Corn Chowder with Red Pepper Oil,
    137
Caviar Lentils, 261
Chapin, Henry D., 4
Chard, 88
Cheese; *See also* Mac 'n' Cheese
    Baked Chicken Parmesan with Bright & Chunky
    Marinara, *148*, 149–150

Baked Ziti with Toasted Chickpeas & Squash,
    256, 257
Blue Cheese Dressing, 245
Italian Rice Balls with Red Pepper Oil & Lemon
    Pesto, 78, *79*
Sautéed Tortellini & Sausage with Collard Greens,
    158, *159*
Cherry Jam, 248
Chicken
    Baked Chicken Parmesan with Bright & Chunky
    Marinara, *148*, 149–150
    Chicken & Almond Dumplings, *164*, 165
    Chicken Madras & Yogurt Sauce with Harissa,
    166, *167*, 168
    Chicken Pad Thai, 156, *157*
    chicken stock, 100
    Chopped Chicken Salad with Pickled Onions
    & Radishes, 147, *148*
    Grilled Chicken with Homemade Barbecue Sauce,
    160, *161*, 163
    Kalamata Chicken with New Potatoes, 144, *145*
    Masala Chicken Wrap with Cabbage Slaw, *142*, 143
    Red Chicken with Baked Biriyani, 170, *171*
    Rustic Lemon Chicken, 140, *141*
    Santa Fe Mac 'n' Cheese, *214*, 215
    Sautéed Tortellini & Sausage with Collard Greens,
    158, *159*
    Slow Broth, 222
    Split Chicken with Lemon Garlic Sauce & Roasted
    Vegetables, 154, *155*
Chickpeas
    Baked Ziti with Toasted Chickpeas & Squash,
    256, 257
    Chopped Chicken Salad with Pickled Onions
    & Radishes, 147, *148*
    Falafel with Chunky Cucumber Yogurt Sauce,
    262, *263*
    Pan-Roasted Chickpeas & Summer Vegetables,
    132, *133*
    Toasted Chickpeas with Ghost Pepper Salt, 84, *85*
Chicory coffee, 62
Children
    attachment disorder, 4
    benefits of family meals, 15, 16
    family meal frequency, 13–15
    nurturing, 3, 4
    obesity, 16
Chile & Lime-Spiced Bay Scallops, 108, *109*

Chiles; *See also* Jalapeños
  Coconut Rice Porridge with Adacherri, 115
  Harissa, 168
  Sambal, 196
  Vindaloo Spice Mix, 209
Chilled Black Bean Yogurt Soup, 102, *103*
Chilled Soba with Spicy Red Beans & Poached Eggs,
  254, *255*
Chocolate, 68, 69, 282
Chopped Chicken Salad with Pickled Onions
  & Radishes, 147, *148*
Chowder, 137
Chunky Cucumber Yogurt Sauce, 262
Chutney, 115
Cinnamon Shortbread Cookies with Fresh Jam,
  286, 287–288
Citrus Salad with Yuzu Dressing & Wonton Crisps,
  128, *129*
Classic Hummus, *90*, 91
Coconut Rice Porridge with Adacherri, 115
Cod
  Miso & Maple–Marinated Cod with Sweet
    Pea Risotto, 186, *187*, 188
  Pepper-Crusted Cod with Sambal, 196, *197*
Coffee, Vietnamese-Style, *62, 63*
Collard greens, 158
Comfort foods, 21
Commensality, 11, 12
Community, 7, 13, 20, 41
Cookies
  Cinnamon Shortbread Cookies with Fresh Jam,
    286, 287–288
  PB&J Cookies, *274*, 275
Copernicus, Nicolaus, 8
Corn
  Almond Cornbread with Grilled Stone Fruit,
    280, 281
  Cauliflower & Corn Chowder with Red Pepper Oil,
    136, 137
  Grilled Romaine with Pancetta, Hard-Boiled
    Eggs & Dijon Dressing, 123, *124*, 125
  Guacamole with Beans, *76*, 77
  Santa Fe Mac 'n' Cheese, *214*, 215
Cornichons, 191
Country-Style Hoisin Ribs, *218*, 219
Cucumber
  Chilled Black Bean Yogurt Soup, 102, *103*
  Chunky Cucumber Yogurt Sauce, 262

Grilled Salmon Steak Sandwiches, 184, *185*
  pickled, 191
  Salty Cucumber Lime Soda, *58*, 59
Culture, 3
  diet-health disparities, 17–20
  differences in commensality, 13–16
  individualism versus collectivism, 7, 12, 13
  versus technology, 30–34
  tradition, 2, 11, 30, 34, 40
Curry, mixed bean, *258*, 259

Dark Chocolate Bark with Spiced Pumpkin Seeds,
  282, 283
Diabetes, 20, 36
Diet-health paradox, 17–20
Diets, 18
Dijon Dressing, 123
Disconnectedness, 23, 26, 28, 33, 40
Dressings
  Blue Cheese, 245
  Dijon Dressing, 123
  for Fresh Grapefruit & Avocado Salad, 113
  Lemon Tarragon Dressing, 87
  Mustard Yogurt Dressing, 184
  Red Pepper Sesame Oil Dressing, 127
  Yuzu Dressing, 128
Dried fruit
  Baked Biriyani, 170, *171*
  Baklava, 285
  Chopped Chicken Salad with Pickled Onions &
    Radishes, 147, *148*
  Homemade Granola, 278
  Masala Chicken Wrap with Cabbage Slaw,
    142, 143
  Soda Bread, 237
Dry herbs, 162
Dumplings, almond, 165
Dusting, 182

Eating disorders, 16, 25, 26, 27
Eckersley, Richard, 30
Eggplant & Onion Fried Wild Rice, 266, *267*
Eggs
  Chilled Soba with Spicy Red Beans & Poached
    Eggs, 254, *255*
  Eggplant & Onion Fried Wild Rice, 266, *267*
  Grilled Romaine with Pancetta, Hard-Boiled
    Eggs & Dijon Dressing, 123, *124*, 125

Homemade Egg Pasta with Fresh-Chopped Sauce, *268*, 269
Emotional health, 4, 9, 22, 23

Falafel with Chunky Cucumber Yogurt Sauce, 262, *263*
Family meals, 12, 13–16, 38
Family-style, 20
Farrow, 249
Fast-food dining, 19–20, 22
Fennel Slaw, 251
Fish, *See Salmon; Seafood*
Five-Ring Fever, 5–7
Flank Steak with Torn Heirloom Tomatoes, *232*, 233
Flash pickling, 210
Food; *See also* Nutrition
   eating alone, 25, 26, 32, 33–34
   family-style, 20
   in hierarchy of needs, 2, 3
   how we eat, 18–20
   opposing perspectives on, 40
   quality of, 18
   religious associations, 11
   sharing with others, 11–12, 19, 26, 28, 39
   technocentric versus ethnocentric, 30–34, 35
Framingham Heart Study, 29
French culture, 14–15, 17
French paradox, 17–20
Fresh-Chopped Sauce, 269
Fresh Grapefruit & Avocado Salad, *112*, 113
Fresh Jalapeño Hot Sauce, 215
Fresh Jam, 287, 288
Fresh Spinach Pasta, 152–153
Fresh Tomatillo Sauce, 195
Fresh versus dry ingredients, 162
Fried rice, 266
Fruit; *See also* Dried fruit
   Banana Mousse Dessert, 272, *273*
   Blackened Pork Loin & Pickled Onions with Baked Apples, *207*, 208
   Citrus Salad with Yuzu Dressing & Wonton Crisps, 128, *129*
   Fresh Grapefruit & Avocado Salad, *112*, 113
   Grilled Stone Fruit, *280*, 281
   jams, 191–192, 248, 275, 287, 288
   juice, 59
   Roast Pork Loin with Peach Glaze & White Beans, 216, *217*

Ghost Pepper Salt, 84
Ginger Barbecue Salmon, 198, *199*
Ginger Barbecue Sauce, 198
Girona, Spain, 22, 29
Granola, homemade, 278
Grapefruit, 113
Greens; *See also* Salads
   Bitter Chard on Grilled Bread, 88, *89*
   Falafel with Chunky Cucumber Yogurt Sauce, 262, *263*
   Grilled Salmon Steak Sandwiches, 184, *185*
   Pepper-Crusted Cod with Sambal, 196, *197*
   Sausage, Potato & Kale Soup, 202, 203
   Sautéed Tortellini & Sausage with Collard Greens, 158, *159*
Grilled Bread & Artichokes with Dipping Oil, *72*, *73*–74
Grilled Chicken with Homemade Barbecue Sauce, 160, *161*, 163
Grilled Pork Chops with Kabocha Squash Mash, 204, *205*
Grilled Romaine with Pancetta, Hard-Boiled Eggs & Dijon Dressing, 123, *124*, 125
Grilled Salmon Steak Sandwiches, 184, *185*
Grilled Stone Fruit, 281
Grilled T-Bones with Blue Cheese Dressing & Radicchio Slaw, *244*, 245, 246
Grilling, baking before, 161
Grilling salt, 206
Guacamole with Beans, *76*, 77

Happiness, 26
   as social contagion, 28–29
   versus success, 7, 8–9
Harissa, 168
Harlow, Harry, 3
Health
   diet-health paradox, 17–20
   emotional, 4, 9, 22, 23
   familial care and, 4, 5, 6–7
   isolation and, 3, 7, 23, 25, 33
   loneliness and, 23–25
   relative depravation, 30–31
   wellness versus illness, 29
Herbs, fresh versus dry, 162
Hoisin Sauce, 219
Homemade Barbecue Sauce, 163

Homemade Egg Pasta with Fresh-Chopped Sauce, *268*, 269
Homemade Hot Chocolate, 68, 69
Hot sauce, 215
Human needs, 2, 3–4, 23
Human performance, 2; *See also* Athletic performance
Hummus, 91

Irish Lamb Stew with Guinness & Soda Bread, *236*, 237–238
Iron absorption, 35–36
Italian Rice Balls with Red Pepper Oil & Lemon Pesto, 78, 79

Jalapeños
  Cabbage Slaw, 143
  Chicken Madras & Yogurt Sauce with Harissa, 166, *167*
  Fresh Jalapeño Hot Sauce, 215
  Fresh Tomatillo Sauce, 195
  Kimchee Spiced Salad, *126*, 127
  Roasted Tomato Yogurt Sauce, 172
  Spicy Red Beans & Rice, 118, *119*
Jambalaya, 180, *181*
Jams, 248, 287, 288
Japanese culture, 17, 19–20

Kabocha Squash Mash, 204, 205
Kalamata Chicken with New Potatoes, 144, *145*
Kale, 203
Kimchee Spiced Salad, *126*, 127
Kokology, 31–32
Kombu seaweed, 221, 222
Korean red pepper, 127

Lamb
  Irish Lamb Stew with Guinness & Soda Bread, *236*, 237
  Lamb Chops with Cherry Jam, Farro & Fennel Slaw, *247*, 248–249, *251*
Leeks, 135
Lemon Garlic Sauce, 154
Lemon Hibiscus Iced Tea with Honey, 52, *53*
Lemon Pesto, 80
Lemon Tarragon Dressing, 87
Lentils, caviar, 261
Lobster Mac 'n' Cheese with Fresh Tomatillo Sauce, 193, *194*

Loneliness, 21–26, 28
Loneliness (Moustakas), 23
Lustig, Robert, 36

Mac 'n' Cheese
  Bolognese, *240*, 241
  Lobster, 193
  Santa Fe, *214*, 215
Marinara, 149–150
Masala Chicken Wrap with Cabbage Slaw, *142*, 143
Maslow, Abraham, 2, 3
Meat, *See* Beef; Chicken; Lamb; Pork
Meatballs, turkey, 105
Miso & Maple–Marinated Cod with Sweet Pea Risotto, 186, *187*, 188
Mixed Bean Curry, *258*, 259
Moustakas, Clark, 23
Mumbai Spiced Chai, *54*, 55
Mushrooms
  Chicken Madras & Fresh Yogurt Sauce with Harissa, 166, *167*, 168
  Flank Steak with Torn Heirloom Tomatoes, *232*, 233
  Slow Broth, 222
  Sweet Potato, Pecan & Mushroom "Meatloaf," *264*, 265
  Tuna Mushroom Salad with Lemon Tarragon Dressing, 86, 87
Mussels, 181
Mustard Yogurt Dressing, 184

New potatoes, 144
Noodles, *See* Pasta
Nutrition
  for athletes, 9
  facts, 293–298
  pragmatism versus extremism, 35–39
Nuts
  Baklava, *284*, 285
  Banana Mousse Dessert, 272, *273*
  Cashew Honey Brittle, *276*, 277
  Lemon Pesto, 80
  Olive Oil–Poached Tomato Soup with Walnuts, 110, *111*
  on salads, 106, 113
  Sweet Potato, Pecan & Mushroom "Meatloaf," *264*, 265
  Sweet Potato–Stuffed Wonton Soup, *120*, 121

Oats, 278
Obesity, 16, 20, 25, 36
Oils
  Balsamic Dipping Oil, 73
  basil, 79
  extra-virgin olive oil, 111
  Red Pepper Oil, 78, 137
  Red Pepper Sesame Oil, 127
Olive Oil–Poached Tomato Soup with Walnuts,
  110, *111*
Olympic Training Center, 5, 6, 7
Onions, pickled, 147, 208
Oysters, in jambalaya, 180

Pad thai, chicken, 156, *157*
Pancetta, 123, 125
Pan-Roasted Chickpeas & Summer Vegetables,
  132, *133*
Pasta
  Allen's Ramen, 221–222
  Baked Ziti with Toasted Chickpeas & Squash,
    256, 257
  Chicken Pad Thai, 156, *157*
  Chilled Soba with Spicy Red Beans & Poached
    Eggs, 254, *255*
  Fresh Spinach Pasta, 152–153
  Homemade Egg Pasta with Fresh-Chopped Sauce,
    268, 269
  Lobster Mac 'n' Cheese with Fresh Tomatillo Sauce,
    193, *194*
  Mac 'n' Cheese Bolognese, 240, 241
  Pasta with Maple Carrots & Leeks, *134*, 135
  ramen noodles, 221–222, 224–225
  Santa Fe Mac 'n' Cheese, *214*, 215
  selecting shapes, 194
Pastry, 191
PB&J Cookies, *274*, 275
Pepper-Crusted Cod with Sambal, 196, *197*
Peppers, *See* Bell peppers; Chiles; Jalapeños
Pesto, lemon, 80
Phinney, Taylor, 22, 38, 39
Pickled Onions, 147, 208
Pickled Radishes, 147
Pickling, flash, 210
Pork
  Blackened Pork Loin & Pickled Onions with
    Baked Apples, *207*, 208
  bones in broth, 222

Country-Style Hoisin Ribs, *218*, 219
Grilled Pork Chops with Kabocha Squash Mash,
  204, *205*
pork shoulder, 220
Roast Pork Loin with Peach Glaze & White Beans,
  216, *217*
Santa Fe Mac 'n' Cheese, *214*, 215
Sausage, Potato & Kale Soup, *202*, 203
Spicy Red Beans & Rice, 118, *119*
Stewed Black-Eyed Peas with Salt Pork,
  212, 213
Porridge, *114*, 115
Portion sizes, 18, 19
Potatoes
  Irish Lamb Stew with Guinness & Soda Bread,
    236, 237–238
  Kalamata Chicken with New Potatoes,
    144, *145*
  Sausage, Potato & Kale Soup, *202*, 203
  Sweet Potato, Pecan & Mushroom "Meatloaf,"
    264, 265
  Sweet Potato–Stuffed Wonton Soup, *120*, 121
  Warm German Potato Salad, *130*, 131
Pumpkin seeds, 282

Radicchio Slaw, 246
Radishes, pickled, 147
Radish & Leek Slaw, 233
Ramen noodles, 220, 227
  Allen's Ramen, 221–222
  making fresh, 224–225
Raspberry jam, 288
Red Chicken with Baked Biriyani, 170, *171*
Red Pepper Oil, 78, 137
Red Pepper Sesame Oil Dressing, 127
Ribs, 219
Rice
  Baked Biriyani, 170, *171*
  Baked Jambalaya, 180, *181*
  Coconut Rice Porridge with Adacherri, 115
  Eggplant & Onion Fried Wild Rice, 266, *267*
  Italian Rice Balls with Red Pepper Oil & Lemon
    Pesto, 78, *79*
  Spicy Red Beans & Rice, 118, *119*
Risotto, 186, 188
Roasted Tomato Yogurt Sauce, 172
Roast Pork Loin with Peach Glaze & White Beans,
  216, *217*

Rose hips, 66, 67
Roux, 180, 181
Rustic Lemon Chicken, 140, *141*

Salads
  Chopped Chicken Salad with Pickled Onions, 147, *148*
  Citrus Salad with Yuzu Dressing & Wonton Crisps, 128, *129*
  Fresh Grapefruit & Avocado Salad, *112*, 113
  Grilled Romaine with Pancetta, Hard-Boiled Eggs & Dijon Dressing, 123, *124*, 125
  Kimchee Spiced Salad, *126*, 127
  Torn Bread & Radicchio Salad, 106, *107*
  Tuna Mushroom Salad with Lemon Tarragon Dressing, *86*, 87
  Warm German Potato Salad, *130*, 131
Salmon
  Baked Salmon in Pastry, *190*, 191–192
  Ginger Barbecue Salmon, 198, *199*
  Grilled Salmon Steak Sandwiches, 184, *185*
Salt, for grilling, 206
Salty Cucumber Lime Soda, *58*, 59
Sambal, 196
Santa Fe Mac 'n' Cheese, *214*, 215
Sauces; *See also* Dressings; Jams; Oils
  Adacherri, 115
  Bright & Chunky Marinara, 149–150
  Chunky Cucumber Yogurt Sauce, 262
  Fresh-Chopped Sauce, 269
  Fresh Jalapeño Hot Sauce, 215
  Fresh Tomatillo Sauce, 195
  Ginger Barbecue Sauce, 198
  Harissa, 168
  Hoisin, 219
  Homemade Barbecue Sauce, 163
  Lemon Garlic Sauce, 154
  Lemon Pesto, 80
  Roasted Tomato Yogurt Sauce, 172
  Roux, 180, 181
  Sambal, 196
  Yogurt Sauce, 166
Sausage
  Baked Jambalaya, 180, *181*
  Sausage, Potato & Kale Soup, *202*, 203
  Sautéed Tortellini & Sausage with Collard Greens, 158, *159*
  Spicy Red Beans & Rice, 118, *119*

Sautéed Tortellini & Sausage with Collard Greens, 158, *159*
Seafood; *See also* Salmon
  Baked Jambalaya, 180, *181*
  Broccoli Soup with Smoked Trout & Chives, *116*, 117
  Catfish Piccata, 183
  Chile & Lime-Spiced Bay Scallops, 108, *109*
  dusting, 182
  Lobster Mac 'n' Cheese with Fresh Tomatillo Sauce, 193, *194*
  Miso & Maple–Marinated Cod with Sweet Pea Risotto, 186, *187*, 188
  Pepper-Crusted Cod with Sambal, 196, *197*
Seaweed, 221, 222
Seeds
  Dark Chocolate Bark with Spiced Pumpkin Seeds, 282, *283*
  Harissa, 168
  in salads, 127, 128
  Vindaloo Spice Mix, 209
Sharing of food, 9, 11–12, 19, 41
Shoyu base, 221
Shrimp, in jambalaya, 180
Slaws
  Cabbage Slaw, 143
  Fennel Slaw, 251
  fresh, 250
  Radicchio Slaw, 246
  Radish & Leek Slaw, 233
Slow Broth, 222
Social contagion phenomenon, 28–29
Social fuel, 3–4
Social support, 8, 23, 25
Social surrogacy, 7, 21
Soda Bread, *236*, 237–238
Soup; *See also* Stew; Stock
  Broccoli Soup with Smoked Trout & Chives, *116*, 117
  Cauliflower & Corn Chowder with Red Pepper Oil, 137
  Chilled Black Bean Soup, 102, *103*
  Olive Oil–Poached Tomato Soup with Walnuts, 110, *111*
  Sausage, Potato & Kale Soup, *202*, 203
  Slow Broth, 222
  Soy Ginger Broth, 121
  Sweet Potato–Stuffed Wonton Soup, *120*, 121
  Turkey Meatball & Tomato Soup, *104*, 105

Soy Ginger Broth, 121
Spain, 17, 22, 29
Sparkling Ginger Soda, 64, 65
Spiced Apple Cider, 56, 57
Spice mix, 209
Spicy Red Beans & Rice, 118, 119
Spinach pasta, 151, 152–153
Split Chicken with Lemon Garlic Sauce & Roasted
    Vegetables, 154, 155
Squash, 257, 204, 132
Steak, See Beef
Stew, 243, 237–238
Stewed Black-Eyed Peas with Salt Pork,
    212, 213
Stock, 98–100
Sugar, 36
Sweet Pea Risotto, 186, 188
Sweet Potato, Pecan & Mushroom "Meatloaf,"
    264, 265
Sweet Potato–Stuffed Wonton Soup, 120, 121
Swiss Mountain Herb Tea, 66, 67

Table seating, 1–2
Tea
    Lemon Hibiscus Iced Tea with Honey, 52, 53
    Mumbai Spiced Chai, 54, 55
    Swiss Mountain Herb Tea, 66, 67
Toasted Chickpeas with Ghost Pepper Salt, 84, 85
Tofu, 156
Tomatillos, 195
Tomatoes
    Baked Jambalaya, 180, 181
    Flank Steak with Torn Heirloom Tomatoes, 232, 233
    Irish Lamb Stew with Guinness & Soda Bread,
        236, 237–238
    Mixed Bean Curry, 258, 259
    Olive Oil–Poached Tomato Soup with Walnuts,
        110, 111
    Roasted Tomato Yogurt Sauce, 172
    Turkey Meatball & Tomato Soup, 104, 105
Torn Bread & Radicchio Salad, 106, 107
Tortellini, 158
Trout, 117
Tuna Mushroom Salad with Lemon Tarragon Dressing,
    86, 87
Turkey Meatball & Tomato Soup, 104, 105

United Kingdom, 14

Vegetables; See also under specific name
    Baked Biriyani, 170
    Broccoli Soup with Smoked Trout & Chives, 116, 117
    Cauliflower & Corn Chowder with Red Pepper Oil,
        137
    Pan-Roasted Chickpeas & Summer Vegetables,
        132, 133
    Pasta with Maple Carrots & Leeks, 134, 135
    pickling, 147, 208, 210
    Split Chicken with Lemon Garlic Sauce & Roasted
        Vegetables, 154, 155
    Sweet Pea Risotto, 186, 188
    Vegetable Stock, 100
Vietnamese-Style Coffee, 62, 63
Vindaloo Spice Mix, 209

Warm German Potato Salad, 130, 131
Watermelon Soda with Fresh Mint, 60, 61
Well-being, 4, 23, 29
White Anchovy Toast, 82, 83
Whole foods, 18, 20
Wiggins, Bradley, 34
Winch, Guy, 23
Wonton crisps, 128
Wonton soup, 121
Wraps, chicken, 142, 143

Yogurt
    Baked Salmon in Pastry, 190, 191–192
    Banana Mousse Dessert, 272, 273
    Cauliflower & Corn Chowder with Red Pepper Oil,
        137
    Chicken Madras & Yogurt Sauce with Harissa,
        166, 167, 168
    Chilled Black Bean Yogurt Soup, 102, 103
    Falafel with Chunky Cucumber Yogurt Sauce,
        262, 263
    Masala Chicken Wrap with Cabbage Slaw, 142, 143
    Mustard Yogurt Dressing, 184
    Red Chicken with Baked Biriyani, 170, 171
    Roasted Tomato Yogurt Sauce, 172
    Vietnamese-Style Coffee, 62, 63
Yuzu Dressing, 128

ACKNOWLEDGMENTS

We would like to thank our friends who opened up their kitchens and homes for us to cook and eat together. To Scott Lynes and Bryan Coulthard, thank you for allowing us to take over your house for the full week of food shoots, for your input on the food, and for helping to eat everything exactly as pictured. And thanks to Johnny Horan, who helped Biju cook all these dishes so they could be photographed.

To Jonathan and Emily Power for sharing their beautiful patio at one of our favorite Denver restaurants, The Populist. And thanks to the friends who joined us for dinner there: Jenny Damitio, Coby Derksen, Alex Howes, Christie Lambert, Poss Lambert, and Daimeon Shanks.

To our friends who ate with us at Allen's house: Lentine Alexis, Scott Berryman, Craig Lewis, Taylor Phinney, and Priya Thomas.

To Biju's friends and partners at Little Curry Shop: Dusty Astrom, Chris Fortune, Jeff Frehner, Scott Lynes, Frank Matson, Caiti Rowe, and Todd Stockbauer. And to the staff: Michael Bowman, Diana Coronado, Fabio Flagiello, David Hadley, Mario Hernandez, Victor Hernandez, Larry Hobbs, Gisella Lopez, Heidi Selander, and Josh Sperry. And to our friends who came to eat with us at Biju's Little Curry Shop: Brandon Anderson, Adrian Encalada, Sean Gilligan, T. J. McReynolds, Bjørn Selander, Spence Smith, and Steve Vanica.

To Biju's friends and neighbors in RiNo: the team at Park Burger for feeding us; Jeff Osaka, Ken Wolfe, Ari Stutz, and Brandon Proff for beers.

To the team at Skratch Labs: Nic Aish, Lentine Alexis, Adin Baird, Chad Brantley, Tony Cesolini, Elyse Cosentino, Jason Donald, Mike Duncan, Annie Dwyer, Aaron Foster, Caleb Freeman, Alex Hoese, Jeff Kenyon, Cole Kramer, Ian MacGregor, Jen MacGregor, Shawn Milne, Jon Robichaud, and Jay Peery.

To the photographers: Aaron Colussi and Jeff Nelson.

To the team at VeloPress, without whom this book would never see the light of day: Haley Berry, Ted Costantino, Vicki Hopewell, Renee Jardine, and Dave Trendler.

*Most importantly, to our families—
our moms, dads, brothers, sisters, aunts,
uncles, cousins, nieces, and nephews—who
are at the very heart of our table.*

ABOUT THE AUTHORS

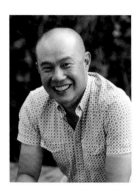

Dr. Allen Lim received his doctorate from the Applied Exercise Science Laboratory in the Department of Integrative Physiology at the University of Colorado under the direction of Dr. William Byrnes. His doctoral work focused on the use of portable power meters to better understand the demands associated with professional cycling. After graduating from the University of Colorado in 2004, Allen worked on the Pro Cycling Tour as a sport scientist and coach for the TIAA-CREF, Slipstream, Garmin, and Radio Shack professional cycling teams.

In 2012, Allen cofounded Skratch Labs (www.skratchlabs.com), a food and beverage company with a mission to provide people with the inspiration, life skills, and products to take better care of themselves and their families. For Allen, the Feed Zone series of cookbooks, which includes *The Feed Zone Cookbook*, *Feed Zone Portables*, and *Feed Zone Table*, is an important part of that mission, helping to give people the basic skills and knowledge to prepare real food from scratch as part of an active lifestyle. When home in Boulder, Colorado, Allen's favorite leisure activities include riding his bike, cooking, and taking naps.

Follow Allen: @skratchlabs

Biju Thomas comes from a big family of cooks who love to eat, entertain, and talk about food. Biju and his family moved from Kerala, India, to Denver when he was 10. From his dad he learned that it's okay for men to cook, and from his mom and his grandmothers he learned how to feed a lot of people quickly without breaking a sweat. He learned from his four older brothers and younger sister that you should eat fast.

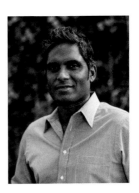

After racing bikes in high school, Biju continued to follow the sport and stay in touch with the guys he knew. He was cooking for a dinner party at Jonathan Vaughters's house when he first met Dr. Allen Lim. In the years since, Biju has cooked for some of cycling's top athletes and teams.

In 2015, Biju and a group of friends launched Biju's Little Curry Shop (www.littlecurryshop.com) in Denver, Colorado. It's a fast-casual Indian restaurant that serves Biju's spin on the made-from-scratch food he grew up eating with his family. When not at the Curry Shop, Biju can be found riding his bike or cooking with his family and friends.

Follow Biju: @bijuthechef, @littlecurryshop

Art direction
Vicki Hopewell

Design
Kevin Roberson

Photography
Aaron Colussi
Pages v, 58, 63, 67, 68, 75 (*bottom left*), 76, 79–80, 82, 85–86, 89–90, 98–99, 101 (*top left, bottom*), 103, 104, 107, 111–112, 114, 116, 119–120, 130, 134, 136, 142, 145–146, 148, 151–153, 155, 157, 159, 161–162, 164, 167–168, 181–182, 185, 189 (*top right, left, bottom right*), 190, 194–195, 197, 199, 202, 205–207, 211–212, 214, 217–218, 232, 234, 236, 239–240, 242, 244, 246–247, 251, 255–256, 258, 260–261, 263, 264, 267, 273–274, 276, 279–280

Kristin Donald
Page xiii (*right*)

Jeff Nelson
Cover and pages v, xiv, 10, 14, 19, 24, 27, 37, 41, 45–47, 50–51, 53, 54, 57, 61, 65, 72, 75 (*top left, top right, bottom right*), 81, 92–95, 101 (*top right, middle*), 109, 122, 124, 126, 129, 133, 141, 169, 171–177, 187, 189 (*bottom left*), 220, 223–229, 268, 283–284, 286, 289, 291–292, 316–317

Jay Peery
Page xiii (*left*)

Photography retouching
Paula Gillen
Elizabeth Riley

Photography locations courtesy of
Biju's Little Curry Shop
Allen Lim
The Populist
Scott Lynes
Skratch Labs

Nutrition analysis
Laura Marzen, RD, LD